AF597551

Shaping the Future with Nutrition

Nestlé Nutrition Institute Workshop Series

Vol. 100

Shaping the Future with Nutrition

September, 2024

Editors

Hania Szajewska Warsaw

Josef Neu Gainesville, FL

Raanan Shamir Petach Tikva

Gary Wong Hong Kong

Andrew Prentice Banjul

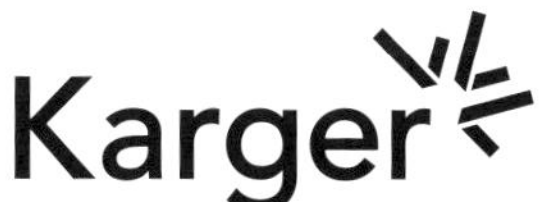

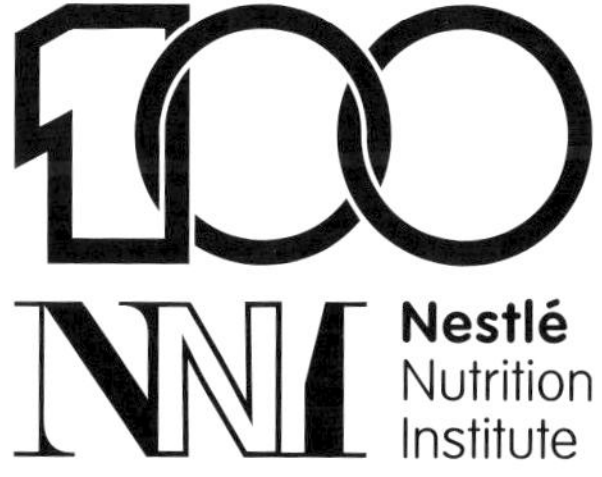

CH-1800 Vevey
S. Karger AG, P.O. Box, CH–4009 Basel (Switzerland) www.karger.com

ISBN 978–3–318–07281–5
e-ISBN 978–3–318–07346–1
ISSN 1664–2147
e-ISSN 1664–2155

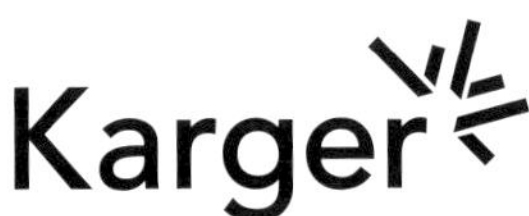

Contents

Session 2: Establishing Good Diet Habits for Optimal Development

Session 3: Addressing Challenges to Feed the Future

Published online: November 15, 2024

Szajewska H, Neu J, Shamir R, Wong G, Prentice AM (eds): Shaping the Future with Nutrition. Nestle Nutr Inst Workshop Ser. Basel, Karger, 2024, vol 100, pp VII–IX (DOI: 10.1159/000540132)

Preface

Our future health may be defined even before we are born. Nestlé Nutrition Institute (NNI) celebrated its 100th workshop in September 2023. The face of nutrition has changed dramatically since the first NNI Workshop in 1980 and this milestone event allowed time to consider just how far our knowledge has advanced in this time. Leading experts in pre- and postnatal nutrition gathered to reflect on the ways in which health is influenced by nutrition, from preconception to childhood, and to explore the role that technology plays in our relationship with food.

Researchers and clinicians gathered to discuss the latest in maternal and child nutrition, the impact of diet on development through childhood and long-term health, as well as the challenges of feeding future generations.

Keynote speaker, Ian MacDonald, discussed the global imbalance between over- and undernutrition and the importance of accurate clinical guidelines for optimizing nutrition for mother and baby through pregnancy and beyond. Malnutrition, whether through over- or undernutrition, is complex and requires education and intervention at many levels, including by government bodies. This can be limited by financial and educational resources, as some countries have access to more funding for investment in early life health and nutrition.

Diet is closely tied to maternal health, particularly ovarian health. This indicates that a woman's diet and lifestyle choices earlier in life can impact fertility and their infant's health. As the expected lifespan increases, some women are having children later in life. In contrast, many young mothers worldwide may still be in the midst of their own development, making them susceptible to nutritional deficiencies. Optimizing nutrition for younger and older mothers is key to support maternal and child health before, during, and after pregnancy.

Alongside the fundamentals of maternal and child nutrition, speakers also looked at some of the difficulties that may be encountered throughout early life, such as feeding difficulties that can impact physical and cognitive growth. Fortifying foods can offer an attractive solution to ensure that children (and parents) receive adequate micronutrients for health and well-being. Early exploration of different food textures can positively influence a child's eating behaviors.

As we continue to learn more about how early life experiences influence gut health, we uncover more about the links between the gut microbiome and health. This covers the time and type of exposure to food, alongside environmental factors and supplementation with pre-and probiotics. Equally, there is currently no universally accepted definition of a "healthy microbiome". Although it is generally accepted that a more diverse microbiome is associated with better health outcomes at least in adults, this resilient ecosystem may be individualized to certain geographical, cultural, or socioeconomic populations. Therefore, perhaps the focus should be on the first 1,000 days of life and how this sets the trajectory of the microbiome through childhood and beyond.

Gut health is still very much an emerging area of research, so there is an urgent need for clear and consistent studies on this topic to help healthcare professionals and policymakers make informed decisions based on the latest scientific evidence. The growing interest in using next-generation Evidence-Based Medicine methods mirrors this trend. These new approaches allow for the adaptation of clinical trials to better serve the unique needs of various populations, thanks to their flexibility and precision.

Sustainability was also a prominent topic for discussion. There has already been a shift towards more plant-based diets in many countries, meaning that the number of children brought up with flexitarian, vegetarian, or vegan diets is likely to increase over the coming years. This presents challenges due to the potential risk for micronutrient deficiencies, as well as the impact that many agricultural practices have on planetary health. While these diet patterns are chosen for a number of reasons, plant-based diets can be higher in unsaturated fats which promote better cardiovascular and metabolic health in adults.

The Workshop also considered how advancements in technology could be harnessed for nutrition and nutraceuticals, from the use of laboratory-grown cells to produce milk-like products to the use of artificial intelligence (AI) for monitoring and early intervention for preterm infants.

A healthy diet, spanning maternal preconception and pregnancy, in addition to infant and childhood nutrition, lays the foundation for long-term health. The rise in digital technologies means that the face of healthcare is likely to look very different over the coming years. Therefore, there is a need to use the most cutting-edge and innovative approaches to progress nutritional research. The methodologies discussed in the 100th NNI Workshop likely look very different from the 1st Workshop. We hope that this book will be helpful to healthcare professionals, researchers, and anyone interested in learning more about nutrition through the lifespan. We look forward to continuing this journey for the next 100 NNI Workshops.

Prof. Hania Szajewska
Department of Paediatrics, The Medical University of Warsaw
Warsaw, Poland

Prof. Josef Neu
University of Florida
Gainesville, FL, USA

Prof. Raanan Shamir
Institute of Gastroenterology, Nutrition and Liver Diseases, Schneider Children's Medical Center
Petach Tikva, Israel

Prof. Gary Wong
Department of Paediatrics, Chinese University of Hong Kong
Shatin, NT, Hong Kong

Prof. Andrew Prentice
Nutrition & Planetary Health, MRC Unit The Gambia @ LSHTM
Banjul, The Gambia

Published online: November 15, 2024

Szajewska H, Neu J, Shamir R, Wong G, Prentice AM (eds): Shaping the Future with Nutrition. Nestle Nutr Inst Workshop Ser. Basel, Karger, 2024, vol 100, pp X–XI (DOI: 10.1159/000540131)

Foreword

This year marks an historical milestone: the 100th Nestlé Nutrition Institute (NNI) Workshop. As we celebrate it, we've been reflecting on Nestlé's rich history, immense dedication, and tireless efforts in supporting and nurturing the nutrition science community through continuous education. This century stands as a testament to our unwavering commitment to advancing the field of nutrition and embracing continuous learning.

Starting with the publication of the first *Annales Nestlé* in 1942, we have been growing in credibility as a source of scientific nutrition-focused information. Along with the growth of the publication, more major milestones were achieved with the first Nestlé Nutrition Workshop, held in France in 1980. The title of that first workshop was "Maternal Nutrition in Pregnancy: Eating for Two?", reminding us that maternal nutrition – also one of the topics covered within the 100th workshop – was already an important theme back then.

These workshops continued to be held, traveling to various regions across the world and providing better access to nutrition science knowledge in different countries, and also providing the launch pad for the iconic publication series, the NNI "Blue Books".

In 2004 the Nestlé Nutrition Institute was created, which then became a not-for-profit association based in Switzerland in 2010. NNI has a long-lasting commitment to unbiased, reliable nutritional science and education. Further milestones were reached as the organization embraced digital technology, launching a website in 2006 and an app in 2022. NNI stays true to its commitment to empowering healthcare providers and supporting the nutrition science community with more accessible digital innovations.

Fast forward to the 100th NNI Workshop, the overall agenda was focused on shaping the future with nutrition, covering topics from preconception through the first months of life up to school age.

In the first section of the workshop, our speakers looked at the current understanding of the fundamentals of maternal and child nutrition. They explored how an individual's health and well-being are shaped by many factors, from maternal preconception nutrition to mode of birth, infant nutrition with the importance of breastfeeding and human milk research, complementary feeding practices, environmental factors, and more.

The second section examined food dietary habits for optimal development. Speakers highlighted a strong evidence base for the nutritional approach that supports good health, but how in practice there are many challenges to achieving this.

During the third session, speakers discussed research into how the food system has evolved to accommodate the challenges that the global nutrition landscape is going through. This involves the shift to a more plant-based diet to account for sustainability in the diet, as well as new technological advancements to help address current and future issues that may persist.

We hope that this summary of the talks provides some food for thought on the strides we have made in nutrition for the different life stages, and the new strategies and solutions, especially in food technology, we can use to overcome the challenges of feeding the future.

Sara Colombo Mottaz
Global Head of the Nestlé Nutrition Institute

Chairpersons, Speakers and Contributors

Bernadette C. Benitez
Section of Developmental and Behavioral Pediatrics
Department of Pediatrics
Makati Medical Center
2 Amorsolo Street
Makati City 1209 Metro Manila
Philippines
bicbenitez@yahoo.com

Aristea Binia
Metabolic Health Department
Nestlé Institute of Health Sciences
Nestlé Research
Société des Produits Nestlé S.A.
Route du Jorat 57, Vers-chez-les-Blanc
CH–1000 Lausanne 26
Switzerland
aristea.binia@rdls.nestle.com

Shiao-Yng Chan
Department of Obstetrics and Gynaecology
Yong Loo Lin School of Medicine
National University of Singapore
1E Kent Ridge Road, 17 NUHS Tower Block, Level 12
Singapore 119228
Singapore
obgchan@nus.edu.sg

Wayne S. Cutfield
Liggins Institute, University of Auckland
Auckland
New Zealand
w.cutfield@auckland.ac.nz

Shaillay Kumar Dogra
Department of Gastrointestinal Health
Nestlé Institute of Health Sciences,
Nestlé Research
Route du Jorat 57
CH–1000 Lausanne 26
Switzerland
shaillaykumar.dogra@rd.nestle.com

Eslam Tawfik Elbaroudy
Department of Pediatrics, Faculty of Medicine
Suez University
Suez
Egypt
Elbaroudy75@yahoo.com

George Jacob Elizabeth
Department of Pediatrics
Ananthapuri Hospitals & Research Institute
Chaka NH, Bypass
Thiruvananthapuram, Kerala 695024
India
drelizake@gmail.com

Ciarán G. Forde
Sensory Science and Eating Behaviour Group
Division of Human Nutrition and Health
Wageningen University & Research
Stippeneng 4
NL–6708 WE Wageningen
The Netherlands
Ciaran.forde@wur.nl

Keith M. Godfrey
MRC Lifecourse Epidemiology Unit
University of Southampton
Southampton
UK
kmg@mrc.soton.ac.uk

Paula Hallam
Plant Based Kids Ltd
39 Queens Road
Kingston upon Thames KT2 7SL
UK
paula@tinytotsnutrition.co.uk

Zhongwei Huang
Department of Obstetrics and Gynaecology
National University of Singapore
NUHS Tower Block, Level 12, 1E Kent Ridge Road
Singapore 119228
Singapore
obgzwh@nus.edu.sg

David L. Kaplan
Department of Biomedical Engineering
Tufts University
4 Colby Street
Medford, MA 02155
USA
david.kaplan@tufts.edu

Julia K. Keppler
Laboratory of Food Process Engineering
Wageningen University & Research
Bornse Weilanden 9
NL–6708 WG Wageningen
The Netherlands
Julia.keppler@wur.nl

Gibby Koshy
Parkview Family Health Care Centre
Kundara, Kollam, Kerala
India
koshy57@yahoo.co.uk

Marine R.-C. Kraus
Nestlé Institute of Health Sciences
Nestlé Research
Société des Produits Nestlé S.A.
EPFL Innovation Park Bldg H
CH–1015 Lausanne
marine.kraus@rd.nestle.com

Marlou P. Lasschuijt
Sensory Science and Eating Behaviour Group
Division of Human Nutrition and Health
Wageningen University & Research
Stippeneng 4
NL–6708 WE Wageningen
The Netherlands
marlou.lasschuijt@wur.nl

Ian A. Macdonald
School of Life Sciences
University of Nottingham
Nottingham
UK
ian.macdonald393@gmail.com

Giles Major
Department of Gastrointestinal Health
Nestlé Institute of Health Sciences,
Nestlé Research
Route du Jorat 57
CH–1000 Lausanne 26
Switzerland
Giles.major@chuv.ch

Cathriona R. Monnard
Metabolic Health, Nestlé Institute of Health Sciences
EPFL Innovation Park, Building G
CH–1015 Lausanne
Switzerland
Cathriona.Monnard@rd.nestle.com

Sara Colombo Mottaz
Nestlé Nutrition Institute
Lausanne
Switzerland
sara.colombomottaz@nestle.com

Josef Neu
Department of Pediatrics/Division of Neonatology
University of Florida
1600 SW Archer Road
Gainesville, FL 32610
USA
neuj@peds.ulf.edu

Andrew M. Prentice
MRC Unit, The Gambia at London School of Hygiene & Tropical Medicine
Fajara, Banjul
The Gambia
Andrew.Prentice@lshtm.ac.uk

Jose M. Saavedra
Department of Pediatrics
Johns Hopkins University School of Medicine
200 N Wolfe St
Baltimore, MD 21287
USA
jose@saavedra.pe

Raanan Shamir
Intistute of Gastroenterology, Nutrition and Liver Diseases
Schneider Children's Medical Center
14 Kaplan St.
Petach Tikva 49202
Israel
raanan@shamirmd.com

Norbert Sprenger
Gastrointestinal Health Department
Nestlé Institute of Health Sciences
Route du Jorat 57, Vers-chez-les-Blanc
CH–1000 Lausanne 26
Switzerland
Norbert.Sprenger@rdls.nestle.com

Hania Szajewska
Department of Paediatrics
Medical University of Warsaw
Żwirki i Wigury 63A
PL–02-091 Warsaw
Poland
szajewska@gmail.com

Eline M. van der Beek
Nestlé Institute of Health Sciences
Nestlé Research
Société des Produits Nestlé S.A.
6 S.A., Route du Jorat 57,
Vers-chez-les-Blanc
CH–1000 Lausanne 26
Switzerland
Eline.vanderBeek@rd.nestle.com

Jens Walter
APC Microbiome Ireland, School of Microbiology, and
Department of Medicine, University College Cork – National University of Ireland
Cork, T12 YT20
Ireland
jenswalter@ucc.ie

Gary Wong
Department of Paediatrics
Chinese University of Hong Kong
Shatin, NT
Hong Kong SAR, China
wingkinwong@cuhk.edu.hk

Keynote Lecture

Published online: November 15, 2024

Szajewska H, Neu J, Shamir R, Wong G, Prentice AM (eds): Shaping the Future with Nutrition. Nestle Nutr Inst Workshop Ser. Basel, Karger, 2024, vol 100, pp 1 15 (DOI: 10.1159/000540138)

Achievements, Challenges, and Future Direction in Early Life Nutrition

Ian A. Macdonald[a] Eline M. van der Beek[b,c] Aristea Binia[d]

[a]Emeritus Professor of Metabolic Physiology, School of Life Sciences, University of Nottingham, Nottingham, UK; [b]Head of Nestlé Institute of Health Sciences, Nestlé Research, Société des Produits Nestlé S.A., Lausanne, Switzerland; [c]Department of Pediatrics, University Medical Centre Groningen, University of Groningen, Groningen, The Netherlands; [d]Head of Metabolic Health Department, Nestlé Institute of Health Sciences, Nestlé Research, Société des Produits Nestlé S.A., Lausanne, Switzerland

Abstract

Malnutrition is present in most countries of the world. This ranges from general undernutrition due to insufficient food, or poor-quality diets low in some essential nutrients, to overnutrition and obesity with energy-rich but nutrient-poor diets. The fundamental aim of dietary recommendations is to prevent deficiency diseases, and the assumptions which underpin these recommendations need to be understood when considering what advice to give to the general public or individual patients. This is particularly relevant in early life as the nutritional state and dietary intake of the mother are of major importance for both her and her baby's health. There is a particular concern with pregnancy in teenage women, as they are still likely to be growing and have different nutrient requirements compared to older women. There is now evidence of beneficial effects for both the mother and baby of supplementation of the mother's diet in those with a low nutritional status. For infants, early gut microbiome development is supported by human milk components (including oligosaccharides) and the reported health benefits are of growing interest and offer potential areas for future developments. Yet, the increasing overweight and obesity in children are a serious concern, in both developed and developing economies. Considerations of the achievements, challenges, and future directions of early life nutrition need to be addressed in a global environment in which every country in the world is experiencing some form of malnutrition. The term malnutrition encompasses a number of different scenarios ranging from undernutrition, which encompasses an inadequate nutrient intake in a diet with a low level of diversity, up to overnutrition where there is an excess of energy intake in a diet which is predominantly composed of nutrient-poor foods. The major feature of malnutrition is that there is micronutrient inadequacy, and even deficiency, which is particularly concerning in early life. The present chapter will consider the major achievements and future challenges in relation to achieving optimal nutrition in early life as well as in older children. Clearly, when considering nutrition in children, it is important to also consider the nutritional state of women before, during, and after pregnancy, as this can have a major impact on the fetus and young child. Before considering these issues in detail, this chapter will begin by addressing the basis on which nutritional recommendations are founded and the challenges that have to be met in getting novel recommendations approved by the appropriate authorities.

Overview of Dietary Requirements and Recommendations

It is well established that diet, nutrition, and lifestyle contribute to health across the life stages. All countries of the world have at least one of the following problems, childhood stunting, anemia in adult women, and overweight in adult women, which all have the potential to have negative effects on infant and child growth and development [1, 2]. Inadequate dietary diversity, poor nutritional status, and an inappropriate lifestyle can be detrimental in both the short and long term. However, health is more than just the absence of disease, and a healthy diet, nutrition, and lifestyle are needed to achieve optimal growth and development, physiological and psychological functions, and to actively promote wellbeing. An ongoing challenge is the need to reliably define wellbeing and measure the beneficial effects that diet, nutrition, and lifestyle have on wellbeing. With respect to disease, there is a major role for diet and nutrition as part of therapeutics in a wide range of illnesses, and public health nutrition has a major part to play in preventing ill health in the population.

There are at least three different components which can contribute to meeting the nutritional demands of an individual: the stores or reserves of nutrients within the body (e.g., fat-soluble vitamins present in the liver and adipose tissue), metabolic transformations of precursors consumed in the diet to active micronutrients (e.g., beta-carotenes being transformed into retinol), and the supply of the nutrient in the diet. If someone is well nourished with adequate stores/reserves and has the metabolic capacity to transform precursors to nutrients in the body, then the dietary changes needed in conditions, such as pregnancy, are relatively minor. But if the woman is poorly nourished with low levels of nutrient stores/reserves, then the dietary needs are much more substantial.

The dietary recommendations produced by public health bodies or other regulators in most countries are designed to prevent deficiency diseases in all age groups, to achieve optimal growth and development in childhood and adolescence, and to maintain health in adulthood. These recommendations include the Dietary Reference Values (DRVs) in the UK, the Dietary Reference Intakes (DRIs) in the US, and the Reference Dietary Intakes or Amounts (RDIs/RDAs) in some other countries. In many cases, the recommendations were made 20–30 years ago, being based on relatively short-term randomized controlled trials, with markers of health as the outcomes, or longer-term prospective cohort studies using health outcomes as the objective markers. The recommendations for individual nutrients have been developed for specific groups of people (e.g., age, sex, and ethnicity); they are based on normal demands in health (not disease states or illness), assume that all other nutrient requirements are being met, and relate to dietary intakes not intravenous nutrition. For many of the nutrients, the recommendations are based on observations of actual requirements for a range of people which fit a normal distribution. Using such data, the recommendation is then set at 97% of the range of intakes for nutrients, such as protein and some of the micronutrients (but not energy), acknowledging that this will exceed the actual requirements of most of the population but that there is little likelihood that this could lead to problems of excess intake.

Although most of the nutrient recommendations were made 20–30 years ago, there are some examples where changes have been made relatively recently. One such example is the recommended dietary fiber intake in the UK. In 2015, the UK Scientific Advisory Committee on Nutrition published a report on carbohydrates and health which substantially increased the recommended intake of fiber [3]. The recommendation to increase adult dietary fiber intake from approximately 14 g/day to 30 g/day was based on evidence from a series of prospective cohort studies, with colorectal disease or cardiovascular disease outcomes. For the first time in the UK, there was also a recommended fiber intake for children which varied by age. Clearly, the disease outcomes used to make the recommendations for adults were not applicable to children, so the committee based the fiber recommendations on the energy recommendations for children relative to adults. When nutritional recommendations are based on expert opinion rather than specific experimental evidence, it should be recognized that there is a potential for some inaccuracy.

The established dietary recommendations are somewhat limited, as they do not include all the potential components of the diet (e.g., phytochemicals, including polyphenols); they do not adequately cover the variations in requirements between individuals and ethnic groups and/or driven by the environment, and they focus mainly on preventing undernutrition without paying much attention to the increasing problem of overnutrition. It is now clear that micronutrient inadequacy exists across a wide range of people around the world. This includes people with obesity who consume a diet of low nutritional quality [4]. Increasing the consumption of plant-based foods or adopting vegetarian and vegan diets may also require the careful consideration of nutritional adequacy, especially when considering specific groups, like children and adolescents. Although the evidence investigating the possible associations between plant-based diets and health outcomes is scarce, common dietary inadequacies associated with plant-enriched diets include protein, iron, vitamin D, calcium, omega-3 fatty acids, vitamin B12, and iodine [5, 6]. It is worth noting that in women consuming vegan and vegetarian diets, there is reduced iodine availability in the mother's breast milk [7]. Whether this increases the risk of impaired child growth and brain development needs to be investigated. It should also be recognized that the evidence base needed to change the current recommendations and to add new "nutrients" or adapt to specific diet patterns is substantial in most countries.

Mothers and Babies

Growing evidence indicates that the vulnerability to noncommunicable diseases (NCDs) later in life is largely set during the first 1,000 days, the period from conception until 2 years of age [8]. Human epidemiological and preclinical model data have convincingly shown that nutrition and other environmental stimuli influence developmental pathways and can induce permanent changes in metabolism and chronic disease susceptibility during this critical period of prenatal and postnatal mammalian development [9]. An adequate nutrition status before conception has considerable promise for health and human capital in this and in the next generation [10]. Although nutritional interventions may only induce subtle changes in the developmental path, these have great potential to reduce later chronic disease risk compared to late interventions for the current and subsequent generations, especially for female offspring, given the fact that the pool of oocytes that harbors the next generation is already present when she is conceived.

Many women do, however, not start their pregnancy in good health or nutrition status. Although undernutrition is still common in some parts of the world, today more and more women enter pregnancy overweight or obese in both low- as well as middle- and high-income countries [11]. Today, obesity and diabetes are global epidemics and are increasingly prevalent in women of reproductive age. Overweight women with a short stature as a consequence of suboptimal nutrition during their own development, may carry the greatest risks for their offspring. The combination of being overweight and a short stature increases the risk of pregnancy complications, such as gestational diabetes [12], which is associated with a higher risk of caesarean section [13] and predicts a higher risk of developing type 2 diabetes during the postpartum period [14].

All forms of malnutrition, including unbalanced diets, increase the risk of nutrient deficiencies and are associated with an increased risk of adverse pregnancy outcomes and long-term health risks for the mother and child [10]. Adolescent girls and women of reproductive age (aged 15–49 years), pregnant and lactating women, and young children are particularly susceptible to the effects of micronutrient malnutrition due to their high requirements. Teenage pregnancies are a particular nutritional risk, given that the body is still under development [10]. A recent pooled analysis, reviewing individual-level biomarker data for the micronutrient status from nationally representative and population-based representative surveys indicated a global prevalence of deficiency of one or more micronutrients, specifically iron, zinc, and folate, to be around 69% among nonpregnant women of reproductive age, equivalent to 1.2 billion women of reproductive age worldwide. Over half (57%) of these women live in East Asia and the Pacific [15].

A varied and healthy diet is a prerequisite to ensure adequate nutrient intake. Pregnancy, however, comes with additional nutrient requirements that are highly specific and not easily met without making serious adjustments in the diet. Although RDAs for some nutrients may not differ than those set for non-pregnant women, like for vitamin D and vitamin E, the recommendations for other nutrients can be up to ~50% higher during pregnancy [16]. For instance, iron, folate, iodide, and vitamin B6 requirements are higher to meet the increased maternal needs, driven by the metabolic and physiological adaptation of the body to pregnancy, as well as the placental and fetal requirements for growth and development (Fig. 1). The diet together with the maternal reserves and metabolic adaptations determine the nutrient supply to both the mother and fetus/infant during pregnancy and lactation. A failure to establish energy and nutrient reserves or competing demands may compromise the supply and affect maternal as well as offspring outcomes.

Nutritional survey data indeed confirm that the diets of many pregnant and lactating women are often nutritionally unbalanced and do not meet local nutritional guidelines and recommendations. A survey conducted among Australian pregnant women showed that the majority of pregnant women in Australia perceive their diets to be healthy [17]. However, they do not consume

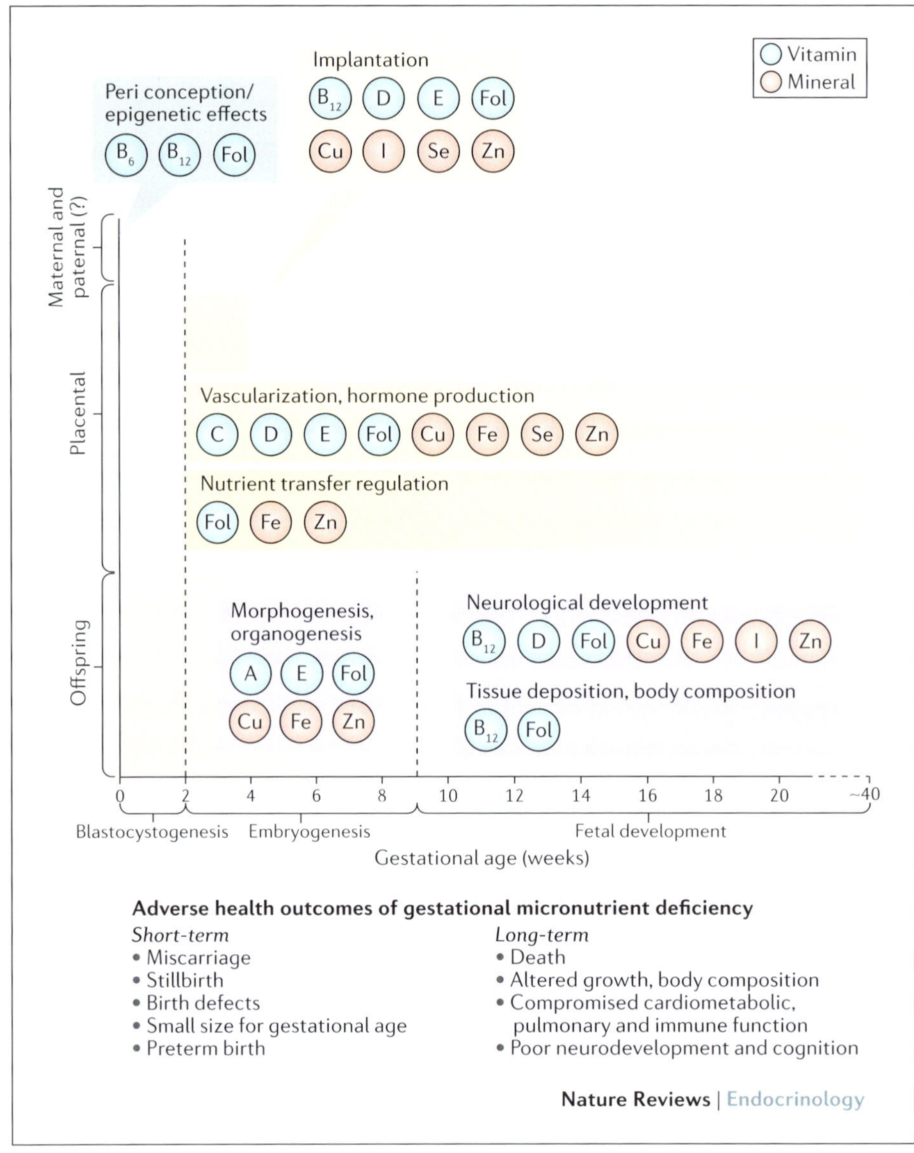

Fig. 1. The function and timing of micronutrients that affect outcomes in offspring. Insights on micronutrient function are primarily derived from reviews of data from in vitro studies, experimental animal models, observational data in human studies and a limited number of trials that have explored metabolic mechanisms and outcomes. The relevant time of action and the function of micronutrients are depicted, but the accumulation of fetal micronutrient stores, generally dependent on the status of the mother, is not. The availability of fetal micronutrient stores to support growth and developmental processes into infancy and beyond is, therefore, an implied pathway. Fol, folate. Reproduced with permission from Gernand et al. [16].

the recommended daily servings from the five major food groups; only 56% met the recommendations for fruits, 29% met those set for dairy, less than 10% met the recommendations for the other core food groups, and none of the women met the recommendations for all five food groups.

In addition, obesity among pregnant women is becoming one of the most important women's health issues worldwide [11]. Maternal obesity is associated with an increased risk of pregnancy complications, such as gestational diabetes mellitus (GDM). GDM currently affects between 6 and 15% of all pregnancies worldwide and is diagnosed in almost 1 out of 4 pregnancies in South East Asia. Both mothers with GDM and their offspring are at an increased risk of short- and longer-term complications, such as the development of type 2 diabetes [18–20].

GDM, defined as glucose intolerance, first diagnosed during pregnancy, develops from the inability of the mother's pancreas to cope with the greater insulin demand [21]. The normal physiological adaptation in insulin secretion driven by changes in insulin sensitivity under the influence of placental hormones serves to maintain an adequate nutrient supply to the growing fetus. The increased supply of glucose, amino acids, and fatty acids that occurs as a consequence of GDM drives faster growth of the fetus, increasing the risk of a high birth weight and neonatal complications [20]. The problem is, however, not restricted to women having a GDM diagnosis. The results of the HAPO study convincingly showed that circulating glucose levels and adverse outcomes is linear, and the more severe the hyperglycemic state, the more severe the consequences will be [22, 23].

Although the currently available evidence favors actions directed at controlling prepregnancy weight and preventing GDM, adequate dietary guidance once GDM is diagnosed, is crucial. Medical nutrition therapy (MNT) is considered to be the first line of treatment for GDM [23]. The dietary advice should be designed to achieve glycemic control and, yet, meet the minimum nutrient requirements for pregnancy. Given the large cultural differences in dietary habits and individual differences driven by a woman's body weight and physical activity, there is currently no universally recommended approach. A pooled analysis of the limited evidence from dietary intervention studies showed that dietary management after the GDM diagnosis resulted in a decrease in both fasting and postprandial glucose, a lower need for medical treatment as well as a lower infant birth weight, and decreased macrosomia rates [24]. However, further assessment of the data in the control arms of these studies clearly indicated that the effectiveness of the intervention was dependent on the background diet [25]. It is of particular interest that the differences in the carbohydrate contribution to the total macronutrient intake impacted the effect size.

To develop meaningful innovations, it is crucial to improve our understanding of the health and nutritional reality of the target populations. Women who have a better nutritional status at the time they conceive are better able to meet the demands imposed by pregnancy and tend to have more successful pregnancy outcomes. Food fortification, where one or more essential nutrients are added to a food to prevent or correct a demonstrated deficiency, can be an effective way to improve nutritional adequacy. However, given the rapid increase in the needs of specific (micro)nutrients over the course of pregnancy, supplementation has shown to be an effective way to improve the nutrient status [10]. Although dietary habits and food availability can differ substantially between regions, it is possible to provide guidance toward an overall diet that is healthy and to identify the aspects that are unhealthy. Healthy diets must include foods with a high nutrient density (high nutrient value per calorie), such as pulses, legumes, vegetables, and fruits, and limit those that are energy rich but nutrient poor, such as sweets, sugar-sweetened beverages, and saturated fats. A reduction of total fat is not a prerequisite of a healthy diet, but the ratio of unsaturated (mono- and polyunsaturated) to saturated fats should be high; synthetic trans fats should be avoided altogether.

Notably, both changing dietary habits as well as changes in agriculture and our food production over the past decades have considerably influenced the fatty acid composition of our dietary fat intake [26]. Since the 1960s, dietary recommendations have been steered toward a decrease in saturated fat intake by the substitution of dairy fats for vegetable oils, mostly high in *n*-6 polyunsaturated fatty acids (PUFAs) and low in *n*-3 PUFAs. In addition, significant changes in animal feeds and the food chain have been introduced, driving an excess in omega-6 intake, which has been hypothesized to be linked to increased obesity risk [26, 27]. These changes in the dietary fat composition have also affected the fatty acid composition of breast milk [26].

Fatty acids obtained through the metabolism of dietary fats as well as by direct dietary intake are known not only as energy sources for the body but also as major structural and bioactive components maintaining normal cellular functions. The World Health Organization recommends a minimum intake of 300 mg of *n*-3 long-chain PUFAs per day and up to 1,000 mg, during pregnancy and lactation, respectively. Despite the common use of over-the-counter supplements containing 200 mg of docosahexaenoic acid (DHA, one of the main *n*-3 long-chain PUFAs) in many parts of the world [28, 29], the median intake is no more than 1/3 of this recommendation. DHA supplementation has been associated with improved pregnancy outcomes and specifically reduced risk of early preterm birth (<34 weeks) [30]. The exact dose associated with the reduced risk of preterm birth, however, is unknown, while women with a low baseline nutritional status may benefit the most [31, 32]. Future clinical trials incorporating screening for the nutritional status would elucidate the regime for DHA supplementation to deliver health benefits while mitigating the risk of any adverse effects.

Human milk is the optimal food for growing infants. Supporting the maternal nutritional status during lactation should be the first line approach to indirectly provide to the infants the necessary nutrients for their growth and development, adapted per life and/or physiological status. Human milk substitutes follow and adhere to the Codex Alimentarius international food standards and other global and national authoritative bodies to deliver the necessary nutritional requirements of infants. Latest research on human milk oligosaccharides (HMOs), a group of prebiotic-like carbohydrates abundantly present in human milk but not affected by the maternal diet, has shown that they are associated with increased protection against infections, immunity, and neurodevelopment as well as the development of the early life gut microbiome [33]. The capacity of the infant microbiome to utilize HMOs has been associated with certain beneficial effects, such as immune competence and bone development. Specifically, the *Bifidobacterium* species can only use HMOs as substrates in contrast to the *Bacteroides* species, and HMOs appear to provide a selective advantage to the *Bifidobacterium* species, postulating toward an ecologically beneficial coevolution between the microbiome and the host [34]. A recent publication reported the identification of a novel distinct *Bifidobacterium* longum clade during weaning in a population of exclusively breast-fed infants from Bangladesh [35]. The novel *Bifidobacterium* longum clade is equipped with enzymes that can utilize both milk and food substrates and produces metabolites implicated in infant health outcomes, emphasizing the probable codependence between the diet and the microbiome during early development.

Another compelling example of how the diet can modify a key development process in early life is provided by a recent clinical study testing the effects of a blend of DHA, arachidonic acid (ARA), iron, vitamin B12, folic acid, and sphingomyelin from a uniquely processed whey protein concentrate enriched in alpha-lactalbumin and phospholipids compared with a control formulation on myelination. The double-blind randomized controlled trial lasted for 12 months, starting at the first month of life, and the children were followed for 12 additional months ($N = 66$). A significantly higher volume and rate of myelination were observed in the investigational compared to the control group at 6, 12, 18, and 24 months of life as assessed through neuroimaging (magnetic resonance imaging, MRI). Additional observations were a significantly higher gray matter volume at 24 months, reduced number of night awakenings at 6 months and increased day sleep at 12 months, and reduced social fearfulness at 24 months in the investigational compared to the control group [36].

The journey of optimizing health and nutrition for infants has two cornerstones: optimal and appropriate maternal nutrition and a deeper understanding of human milk. Recent methodical advances enable the characterization of human milk qualitatively and quantitatively, as well as functionally. Moving beyond a simple catalog of nutrients toward functional structures or networks of nutrients codelivered to the infant gut, while encompassing bioactive molecules is a step forward. Global reference values for both maternal and infant nutrition need to be adapted to subpopulations and stages of development. Testing how targeted maternal intervention can impact the milk composition and infant development, thereafter, needs to be expanded into region-specific approaches and infant populations with defined needs (e.g., suboptimal growth and compromised immune responses). The clinical translation of research findings needs to ultimately fulfill the refined nutritional needs for mothers during pregnancy and the lactation stage, enable the development of safe and efficacious human milk substitutes as well as the optimized use of donor human milk, and finally promote further breastfeeding and lactation.

Overnutrition in Children after Toddlerhood

There is a growing concern about the rise in overweight and obesity in children in many countries. In England, there has been a national child measurement program in school children in the first class in primary school (aged 5 years) and the final year of primary school (aged 11 years) since 2006. Child obesity was defined on the basis of BMI ≥95th centile of the UK90 growth reference, and deprivation deciles were assigned to the child's area of residence using the Index of Multiple Deprivation 2010. In 5-year-old children, the prevalence of obesity was around 7% in children from the least deprived areas in 2006 compared to 12% in the most deprived areas. By 2011, the obesity prevalence had fallen to 6% in the least deprived areas but was maintained at 12% in the most deprived ones. By 2018, the overall obesity prevalence in 5-year-old children was 9.7%, with those in the most deprived areas having more than double the prevalence of that of the children in the least deprived areas. Similar patterns of obesity prevalence in relation to social deprivation were observed in 11-year-old children but the actual prevalence was more than twice that seen in the younger children, i.e., over 20% of 11-year-old children were obese, with a higher obesity prevalence in boys in both age groups [37]. The problem of childhood obesity in England has been recognized for almost 20 years but it is not improving. Clearly, innovative approaches are needed, with input from multiple stakeholders.

Liver Glycogen Stores in Children

The brain volume in children is a higher proportion of body weight than that in adults. The brain's primary metabolic fuel is glucose, and there is a need for a higher relative rate of glucose supply in young children to maintain an optimal brain function. During an overnight fast, the supply of glucose to the brain is derived from the stores of glycogen in the liver, together with the synthesis of glucose (gluconeogenesis) from lactate, glycerol, and some amino acids, which primarily occurs in the liver. The liver glycogen store is, thus, likely to be depleted during an overnight fast, and the child will need to ingest carbohydrate in the morning to initially prevent further depletion of liver glycogen and possibly increase the levels to reverse the effect of the overnight fast. A recent study in children aged 8–12 years used magnetic resonance imaging (MRI) to measure the liver volume and magnetic resonance spectroscopy (MRS) to measure the liver glycogen concentration. Measurements were made in the evening, 3 h after a standardized evening meal, and at 08:00 the following morning immediately before ingesting either a mixed nutrient malt drink (containing 402 kJ and 15.6 g of carbohydrates) or water, with repeat MRI and MRS measurements at hourly intervals for 4 h after the drinks [38]. The overnight fast was accompanied by a reduction of 24.7% in the liver glycogen, which was similar to the 28% reduction seen in adults in a separate study [39]. The absolute concentrations seen in children after an overnight fast (approximately 500 mmol/L) were substantially higher than the overnight fasted values in adults (approximately 300 mmol/L) [40]. When the children consumed the control drink (water), their liver glycogen continued to fall, by another 150 mmol/L over 4 h. By contrast, the carbohydrate drink prevented a further fall in glycogen for the first 2 h before the level began to fall at a similar rate to that seen after water. Further studies are needed to establish the amount of carbohydrates needed to replenish the liver glycogen stores after an overnight fast in children and to assess the impact this might have on the physical and cognitive performance. It is clearly possible that a progressive reduction in the liver glycogen over the morning could impair the supply of glucose to the brain, which could have important implications for learning.

Conclusions and Future Challenges

The major issues to be addressed going forward are illustrated in Figure 2. A particular focus should be given to the following:

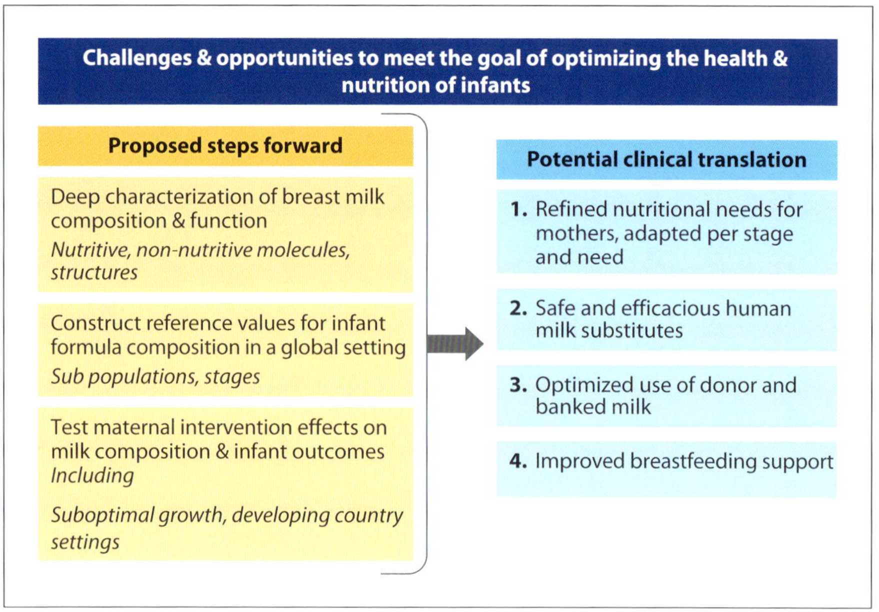

Fig. 2. Challenges and opportunities for early life nutrition.

1. Testing how targeted maternal intervention can impact the milk composition and infant development, thereafter, needs to be expanded into a region-specific approach and infant populations with defined needs (e.g., suboptimal growth and compromised immune responses). It will also be important to further identify the relevance of nutrient-dense foods during weaning and to ensure that the overall nutritional quality of the diet is adapted to meet the nutritional needs.
2. There is a high prevalence of one or more micronutrient deficiencies across geographies in preschool children. It will be important to identify vulnerable groups/populations for intervention either via nutrient-dense foods or supplements.
3. It is clear that the nutritional quality of both fats and carbohydrates is of major importance for the developing and growing child and more attention should be focused on dietary fats and carbohydrates.
4. Obesity and being overweight in the mother before and during pregnancy impose a health burden on both the mother and child as it can compromise the adequate nutritional status and lead to obesity in the child. It is now clear that childhood obesity is a major problem in many developed economies and multiple stakeholders should be involved in addressing this problem.
5. The increasing number of demonstrations of the potential health benefits of prebiotics and probiotics are of great interest. However, before this can be converted into new nutritional recommendations or health claims, we need evidence that they are essential for children's health.

6. There is an increasing interest in plant-based diets and their potential health benefits, especially in adults. Clearly, this may also be of benefit for the growing child, but it will be important to ensure that such diets have adequate amounts of micronutrients, such as vitamin B12, iron, and zinc. However, many meat-based diets have other dietary limitations and so greater attention needs to be focused on the nutritional adequacy of the diets we feed our children, with the appropriate use of fortification or supplementation when needed [38].

Conflict of Interest Statement

Ian Macdonald was a Scientific Director of the Nestle Institute of Health Sciences; an employee of Nestle Research, from August 2020 to August 2022; and is now an Emeritus Professor at the University of Nottingham.

Eline van der Beek is the Director of the Nestle Institute of Health Sciences, and Aristea Binia is the Head of the Metabolic Health Department in the Nestle Institute of Health Sciences.

The opinions expressed in this article are from the authors alone.

There was no additional funding obtained for the preparation of this manuscript with the authors undertaking its preparation as part of their duties at Nestlé Research.

Author Contributions

All authors contributed to the writing of this article and all have read and approved the final version.

References

1 Global Nutrition Report; 2018. https://globalnutritionreport.org/0b98fb.

2 Prentice AM. The triple burden of malnutrition in the era of globalization. Nestle Nutr Inst Workshop Ser. In Rogacion JM, editors. Interactions of nutrition: retracing yesterday, redefining tomorrow. 97th Nestle Nutrition Institute Workshop, June 2022. Nestle Nutr Inst Workshop Ser. Basel: Karger, 2023. Vol. 97, p. 51–61. https://doi.org/10.1159/000529005.

3 SACN. Carbohydrates and health; 2015. Published for Public Health England under licence from the Controller of Her Majesty's Stationery Office. ISBN: 978 0 11 708284 7. Printed in the UK by The Stationery Office Limited.

4 Astrup A, Bugel S. Overfed but undernourished: recognizing nutritional inadequacies/deficiencies in patients with overweight or obesity. Int J Obes. 2019;43(2):219–32. https://doi.org/10.1038/s41366-018-0143-9.

5 Sebastiani G, Barbero AH, Borras-Novell, Casanova MA, Aldecoa-Bilbao V, Andreu-Fernandez V, et al. The effects of vegetarian and vegan diet during pregnancy on the health of mothers and offspring. Nutrients 2019; 11(3):557. https://doi.org/10.3390/nu11030557.

6 Neufingerl N, Eilander A. Nutrient intake and status in children and adolescents consuming plant-based diets compared to meat-eaters: a systematic review. Nutrients 2023;15(20):4341. https://doi.org/10.3390/nu15204341.

7 Pawlak R, Judd N, Donati GL, Perrin MT. Prevalence and predictors of low breast milk iodine concentration in women following vegan, vegetarian, and omnivore diets. Breastfeed Med. 2023; 18(1):37–42. https://doi.org/10.1089/bfm.2022.0211.

8 Godfrey KM, Gluckman PD, Hanson MA. Developmental origins of metabolic disease: life course and intergenerational perspectives. Trends Endocrinol Metab. 2010;21(4):199–205. https://doi.org/10.1016/j.tem.2009.12.008.

9 Waterland RA, Michels KB. Epigenetic epidemiology of the developmental origins hypothesis. Annu Rev Nutr. 2007;27:363–88. https://doi.org/10.1146/annurev.nutr.27.061406.093705.
10 Hanson MA, Bardsley A, De-Regil LM, Moore SE, Oken E, Poston L, et al. The International Federation of Gynecology and Obstetrics (FIGO) recommendations on adolescent, preconception, and maternal nutrition: "think nutrition first". Int J Gynaecol Obstet. 2015;131(Suppl 4):S213–53. https://doi.org/10.1016/S0020-7292(15)30034-5.
11 Chen C, Xu X, Yan Y. Estimated global overweight and obesity burden in pregnant women based on panel data model. PLoS One. 2018;13(8):e0202183. https://doi.org/10.1371/journal.pone.0202183.
12 Yong HY, Mohd Shariff Z, Mohd Yusof BN, Rejali Z, Tee YYS, Bindels J, et al. Early pregnancy body mass index and gestational weight gain: a mediating or moderating factor for short stature and risk of gestational diabetes mellitus? PLoS One. 2022;17(8):e0272253. https://doi.org/10.1371/journal.pone.0272253.
13 Rahman M, Haque SE, Islam MJ, Chau NH, Adam IF, Haque MN. The double burden of maternal overweight and short stature and the likelihood of cesarean deliveries in South Asia: an analysis of national datasets from Bangladesh, India, Maldives, Nepal, and Pakistan. Birth. 2022;49(4):661–74. https://doi.org/10.1111/birt.12632.
14 Cidade-Rodrigues C, Cunha FM, Chaves C, Castro F, Pereira C, Paredes S, et al. Maternal height as a predictor of glucose intolerance in the postpartum and its relationship with maternal pre-gestational weight. Arch Gynecol Obstet. 2023;307(2):601–8. https://doi.org/10.1007/s00404-022-06809-5.
15 Stevens GA, Beal T, Mbuya MNN, Luo H, Neufeld LM; Global Micronutrient Deficiencies Research Group. Micronutrient deficiencies among preschool-aged children and women of reproductive age worldwide: a pooled analysis of individual-level data from population-representative surveys. Lancet Glob Health. 2022;10(11):e1590–9. https://doi.org/10.1016/S2214-109X(22)00367-9.
16 Gernand AD, Schulze KJ, Stewart CP, West KP Jr, Christian P. Micronutrient deficiencies in pregnancy worldwide: health effects and prevention. Nat Rev Endocrinol. 2016;12(5):274–89. https://doi.org/10.1038/nrendo.2016.37.
17 Malek L, Umberger W, Makrides M, Zhou SJ. Adherence to the Australian dietary guidelines during pregnancy: evidence from a national study. Public Health Nutr. 2016;19(7):1155–63. https://doi.org/10.1017/S1368980015002232.
18 Silverman BL, Rizzo TA, Cho NH, Metzger BE. Long-term effects of the intrauterine environment. The Northwestern University Diabetes in Pregnancy Center. Diabetes Care. 1998;21(Suppl 2):B142–9. PMID: 9704242.
19 Farrar D, Simmonds M, Bryant M, Sheldon TA, Tuffnell D, Golder S, et al. Hyperglycaemia and risk of adverse perinatal outcomes: systematic review and meta-analysis. BMJ. 2016;354:i4694. https://doi.org/10.1136/bmj.i4694.
20 van der Beek EM. Chapter 17 Diabetes in pregnancy: neonatal & childhood complications. In Goulis D, editor. Diabetes in pregnancy. Cham: Springer; 2022, p. 311–34.
21 Marcinkevage JA, Narayan KM. Gestational diabetes mellitus: taking it to heart. Prim Care Diabetes. 2011;5(2):81–8. https://doi.org/10.1016/j.pcd.2010.10.002.
22 HAPO Study Cooperative Research Group; Metzger BE, Lowe LP, Dyer AR, Trimble ER, Chaovarindr U, et al. Hyperglycemia and adverse pregnancy outcomes. N Engl J Med. 2008;358(19):1991–2002. https://doi.org/10.1056/NEJMoa0707943.
23 Metzger BE, Buchanan TA, Coustan DR, de Leiva A, Dunger DB, Hadden DR, et al. Summary and recommendations of the Fifth International Workshop-Conference on Gestational Diabetes Mellitus. Diabetes Care. 2007;30(Suppl 2):S251–60. https://doi.org/10.2337/dc07-s225.
24 Yamamoto JM, Kellett JE, Balsells M, García-Patterson A, Hadar E, Solà I, et al. Gestational diabetes mellitus and diet: a systematic review and meta-analysis of randomized controlled trials examining the impact of modified dietary interventions on maternal glucose control and neonatal birth weight. Diabetes Care. 2018;41(7):1346–61. https://doi.org/10.2337/dc18-0102.
25 García-Patterson A, Balsells M, Yamamoto JM, Kellett JE, Solà I, Gich I, et al. Usual dietary treatment of gestational diabetes mellitus assessed after control diet in randomized controlled trials: subanalysis of a systematic review and meta-analysis. Acta Diabetol. 2019;56(2):237–40. https://doi.org/10.1007/s00592-018-1238-4.
26 Ailhaud G, Massiera F, Weill P, Legrand P, Alessandri JM, Guesnet P. Temporal changes in dietary fats: role of n-6 polyunsaturated fatty acids in excessive adipose tissue development and relationship to obesity. Prog Lipid Res. 2006;45(3):203–36. https://doi.org/10.1016/j.plipres.2006.01.003.
27 Muhlhausler BS, Ailhaud GP. Omega-6 polyunsaturated fatty acids and the early origins of obesity. Curr Opin Endocrinol Diabetes Obes. 2013;20(1):56–61. https://doi.org/10.1097/MED.0b013e32835c1ba7.
28 Meyer BJ, Mann NJ, Lewis JL, Milligan GC, Sinclair AJ, Howe PR. Dietary intakes and food sources of omega-6 and omega-3 polyunsaturated fatty acids. Lipids. 2003;38(4):391–8. https://doi.org/10.1007/s11745-003-1074-0.

29 Nordgren TM, Lyden E, Anderson-Berry A, Hanson C. Omega-3 fatty acid intake of pregnant women and women of childbearing age in the United States: potential for deficiency? Nutrients. 2017;9(3):E197. https://doi.org/10.3390/nu9030197.

30 Middleton P, Gomersall JC, Gould JF, Shepherd E, Olsen SF, Makrides M. Omega-3 fatty acid addition during pregnancy. Cochrane Database Syst Rev. 2018;11:CD003402. https://doi.org/10.1002/14651858.CD003402.pub3.

31 Makrides M, Best K, Yelland L, McPhee A, Zhou S, Quinlivan J, et al. A randomized trial of prenatal n-3 fatty acid supplementation and preterm delivery. N Engl J Med. 2019;381(11):1035–45. https://doi.org/10.1056/NEJMoa1816832.

32 Carlson S, Gajewski BJ, Valentine CJ, Kerling EH, Weiner CP, Cackovic M, et al. Higher dose docosahexaenoic acid supplementation during pregnancy and early preterm birth: a randomised, double-blind, adaptive-design superiority trial. EClinicalMedicine. 2021;36:100905. https://doi.org/10.1016/j.eclinm.2021.100905.

33 Sprenger N, Tytgat HLP, Binia A, Austin S, Singhal A. Biology of human milk oligosaccharides: from basic science to clinical evidence. J Hum Nutr Diet. 2022;35(2):280–99. https://doi.org/10.1111/jhn.12990.

34 Milani C, Turroni F, Duranti S, Lugli GA, Mancabelli L, Ferrario C, et al. Genomics of the genus *Bifidobacterium* reveals species-specific adaptation to the glycan-rich gut environment. Appl Environ Microbiol. 2016;82(4):980–91. https://doi.org/10.1128/AEM.03500-15.

35 Vatanen T, Ang QY, Siegwald L, Sarker SA, Le Roy CI, Duboux S, et al. A distinct clade of *Bifidobacterium longum* in the gut of Bangladeshi children thrives during weaning. Cell. 2022;185(23):P4280–4297.e12. https://doi.org/10.1016/j.cell.2022.10.011.

36 Schneider N, Bruchhage MMK, O'Neill BV, Hartweg M, Tanguy J, Steiner P, et al. A nutrient formulation affects developmental myelination in term infants: a randomized clinical trial. Front Nutr. 2022;9:823893. https://doi.org/10.3389/fnut.2022.823893.

37 The national child measurement programme: trends in child BMI; 2019. https://digital.nhs.uk/data-and-information/publications/statistical/national-child-measurement-programme/2018-19-school-year

38 Horstman AMH, Bawden SJ, Spicer A, Darwish N, Goyer A, Egli L, et al. Liver glycogen stores via ^{13}C magnetic resonance spectroscopy in healthy children: randomized, controlled study. Am J Clin Nutr. 2023;117(4):709–16. https://doi.org/10.1016/j.ajcnut.2023.01.014.

39 Rothman DL, Magnusson I, Katz LD, Shulman RG, Shulman GI. Quantitation of hepatic glycogenolysis and gluconeogenesis in fasting humans with 13C NMR. Science. 1991;254(5031):573–6. https://doi.org/10.1126/science.1948033.

40 Bawden S, Stephenson M, Falcone Y, Lingaya M, Ciampi E, Hunter K, et al. Increased liver fat and glycogen stores after consumption of high versus low glycaemic index food: a randomized crossover study. Diabetes Obes Metab. 2017;19(1):70–7. https://doi.org/10.1111/dom.12784.

Ian A. Macdonald
Emeritus Professor of Metabolic Physiology
School of Life Sciences, University of Nottingham
NG7 2UH, UK
ian.macdonald393@gmail.com

Session 1: Getting the Right Start through Maternal and Child Nutrition

Published online: November 15, 2024

Szajewska H, Neu J, Shamir R, Wong G, Prentice AM (eds): Shaping the Future with Nutrition. Nestle Nutr Inst Workshop Ser. Basel, Karger, 2024, vol 100, pp 16–27 (DOI: 10.1159/000540136)

An Offspring's Health Starts Before Conception and Results of the NiPPeR Randomized Trial

Shiao-Yng Chan[a, b] Wayne S. Cutfield[c, d]
Keith M. Godfrey[e, f] the NiPPeR Study Group

[a]Department of Obstetrics and Gynaecology, Yong Loo Lin School of Medicine, National University of Singapore and National University Health System, Singapore, Singapore; [b]Singapore Institute for Clinical Sciences, Agency for Science, Technology and Research (A*STAR), Singapore, Singapore; [c]Liggins Institute, University of Auckland, Auckland, New Zealand; [d]A Better Start, New Zealand National Science Challenge, Auckland, New Zealand; [e]MRC Lifecourse Epidemiology Unit, University of Southampton, Southampton, UK; [f]NIHR Southampton Biomedical Research Centre, University of Southampton and University Hospital Southampton, NHS Foundation Trust, Southampton, UK

Abstract

Improved maternal nutritional status is hypothesized to promote good pregnancy and infant health outcomes but trial evidence supporting the commencement of nutritional supplementation before conception is sparse. The NiPPeR (*Nutritional Intervention Preconception and During Pregnancy to Maintain Healthy Glucose Metabolism and Offspring Health*) multinational double-blind randomized controlled trial conducted in the United Kingdom, Singapore, and New Zealand tested a nutritional formulation containing myo-inositol, probiotics, and multiple micronutrients (intervention), compared with a standard micronutrient supplement (control), taken at preconception and throughout pregnancy. The primary outcome of gestational glycemia at 28 weeks' gestation showed no difference. However, differences in several prespecified secondary outcomes were notable. The intervention reduced the incidence of preterm delivery particularly those associated with preterm prelabor rupture of membranes, operative delivery for delayed second stage, and major postpartum hemorrhage. It may also shorten time to conception in overweight women, to that similar to nonoverweight/obese

Members of the NiPPeR Study Group authors for the Medline citation are listed in the Acknowledgements.

women. Importantly, the intervention associated with a reduction in the incidence of rapid infant weight gain and high body mass index at 2 years among offspring. Such evidence indicates the potential for preconception maternal nutritional interventions to have appreciable impact in shaping the long-term health of an individual and building resilience against noncommunicable chronic diseases in the future.

Introduction

There is wide consensus that early life events can shape future health and well-being. It is hypothesized that the earlier the exposure to a particular environmental factor the greater the impact on future outcome; small changes in early life can lead to the emergence of significant consequences later, with epigenetic mechanisms thought to play a key role [1].

A new life begins at conception when sperm fertilizes the oocyte. This initial environment within which this new life is formed is determined by both maternal and paternal lifestyle prior to pregnancy in addition to genetic make-up (Fig. 1). These could influence pregnancy events and have consequences for offspring health, including the risk of developing noncommunicable diseases and mental health issues.

The Example of Gestational Glycemia Impact on Offspring

The multinational HAPO (Hyperglycemia and Adverse Pregnancy Outcomes) study [2] demonstrated that higher gestational glycemia is linked to higher clinical risk across a continuum for both the woman and her offspring; even small increases in glycemia can have an appreciable effect including the risk of being born large-for-gestational age and having a high cord blood C-peptide level. A high cord C-peptide concentration has been associated with increased odds of being overweight and displaying the metabolic syndrome in adolescence and adulthood [3, 4]. Furthermore, there is evidence that gestational diabetes is associated with suboptimal breast development antenatally, leading to delayed onset of lactation, reduced breastmilk production [5], and altered breastmilk composition [6]. Breast feeding success may be further compounded by peripartum complications that limit early skin-to-skin time such as emergency cesarean delivery, perineal trauma, and neonatal unit admission, which all occur with increased frequency with higher gestational glycemia [2]. A shorter breastfeeding duration and altered breastmilk composition may also themselves

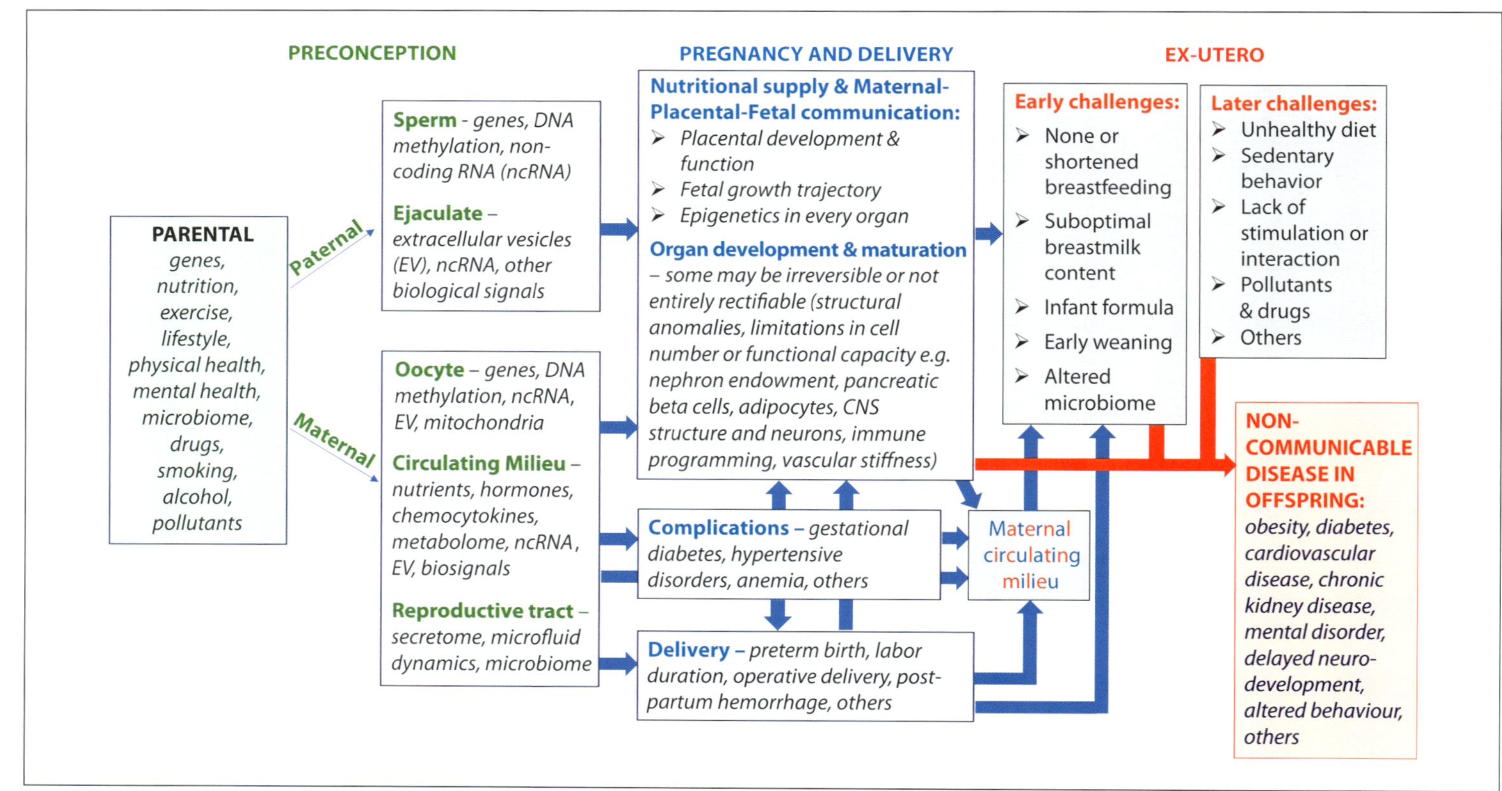

Fig. 1. Influential factors impacting risk of noncommunicable diseases in offspring extends from the preconception phase in both parents, during pregnancy and delivery, and to events and challenges after delivery.

have implications for the development of long-term adverse health in offspring [7], further adding to the effects of exposure to in-utero hyperglycemia, which is already known to associate with offspring cardiometabolic risk [4].

Parental Prepregnancy Health Impacts Offspring Health

Mother-offspring cohort studies show that multiple parental lifestyle risk factors have additive effects on child health [8, 9]; risk increases with each additional risk factor. For example, risk factors for child overweight/obesity include those already present in prepregnancy (e.g., maternal and paternal body mass index [BMI], smoking), in addition to those arising during pregnancy (e.g., excessive gestational weight gain, higher gestational glycemia, vitamin D insufficiency), and postpartum (e.g., shorter breastfeeding duration, early weaning).

Periconception mechanisms operating in gametes and in the reproductive tract are known to be altered by paternal and maternal nutritional status, and this can already begin to affect the early embryo to influence offspring future cardiovascular risk [10]. Paternal obesity and undernutrition have been associated with altered sperm characteristics (decreased motility, DNA damage, altered epigenomic/transcriptomic profiles), seminal fluid composition, and endocrine dysregulation. Similarly, with maternal obesity and undernutrition, there is evidence of disruption in oocyte features (altered metabolite content, mitochondrial damage, endoplasmic reticular stress, epigenetic reprogramming) and in the tubal-utero environment which can be sensed by the preimplantation blastocyst (e.g., nutrients and bioactive factors in reproductive tract fluids) and influence epigenetic/metabolomic reprogramming (e.g., ribosomal biogenesis, compensatory mechanisms).

Appreciation of the extent of this most early influence of preconception parental lifestyle and health on future offspring conditions is mounting as an increasing number of studies of pregnancy interventions have demonstrated more limited effects than expected [11]. After all, epigenetic plasticity peaks around the time of conception. It has led to the postulation that preconception interventions could be more effective in optimizing offspring health trajectories. The immediate effects on the offspring can be subtle earlier in life but such early effects can alter how the person responds to their later environment and lifestyle, including the increasingly diverse array of obesogenic exposures (e.g., high-fat/sugar diets, sedentary behavior). Thus, building resilience *in utero* and in early life could mitigate the impact of later challenges.

Maternal Nutritional Intervention

Many young women across both the developed and developing world are not nutritionally prepared for pregnancy, with a large proportion displaying micronutrient deficiencies and insufficiencies [12]. Of particular note are the rising prevalence of obesity with micronutrient deficiencies [13] and the increasing shift to the less nutrient-dense plant-based diets driven partly by sustainability agendas [14].

Nutrient deficiencies are linked to adverse pregnancy and offspring outcomes. While dietary intervention commencing during pregnancy can correct micronutrient insufficiencies, only some clinical trials have reported lowered pregnancy risks and few have reported improvements in long-term offspring outcomes [15]. It appears that starting nutritional supplementation in pregnancy is insufficient to fundamentally enhance child health [16]. However, evidence supporting maternal nutritional supplementation as a prepregnancy intervention is scarce to date. There is, thus, a need now to build good and specific evidence on the benefit of preconception interventions, the optimal timing of their administration and the population that would derive clear benefit.

NiPPeR Randomized Controlled Trial

To address the sparsity of evidence surrounding the potential benefit of preconception nutritional intervention, the NiPPeR (Nutritional Intervention Preconception and During Pregnancy to Maintain Healthy Glucose Metabolism and Offspring Health) double-blind randomized controlled trial recruited in the United Kingdom (UK), Singapore (SG), and New Zealand (NZ) 1,729 women planning a pregnancy in 2015–2017 [17]. We investigated the combined effects of a nutritional formulation containing myo-inositol, probiotics and multiple micronutrients (intervention), compared with a standard micronutrient supplement (control), taken at preconception and throughout pregnancy. Briefly, supplements for both arms contained folic acid, iron, calcium, iodine and β-carotene; the intervention additionally included myo-inositol, vitamin D, riboflavin, vitamin B6, vitamin B12, zinc, and probiotics (*Lacticaseibacillus rhamnosus* [previously *Lactobacillus rhamnosus*] NCC 4007 [CGMCC 1.3724; LPR] and *Bifidobacterium animalis* sp. lactis NCC 2818 [CNCM I-3446; Bl818]). Women were computer randomized in a 1:1 ratio, with stratification by site and ethnicity to ensure a balanced allocation. Women who were subsequently found to have prepregnancy type 2 diabetes, who underwent assisted conception, and had multiple pregnancies were withdrawn from the trial. Further details of randomization, exclusion and inclusion criteria, doses of supplement components have been previously described [18].

For the vitamins present in the intervention supplement, a notable prevalence of vitamin insufficiency status had previously been reported in the obstetric population at each of our centers. These vitamins have also been reported in observational and preclinical studies to be implicated in insulin resistance, dysglycemia, and increased offspring adiposity [17]. Myo-inositol is a naturally occurring carbohydrate which is a key component of many compounds involved in intracellular signaling and second messenger pathways, in regulating membrane function and acting as hormonal mimics [19]. Myo-inositol promotes insulin sensitivity and antenatal myo-inositol supplementation has been shown to reduce gestational glycemia in earlier studies [20]. Probiotics including *L. rhamnosus* and *B. animalis* have also been reported to lower insulin resistance [21] and gestational glycemia [22]. We had, therefore, hypothesized that the combined effect of all these components would serve to promote optimal glycemic regulation during pregnancy and enhance development of normal offspring adiposity.

NiPPeR Trial Population Characteristics and Primary Outcome

Women planning pregnancy were recruited from the community and were generally healthy. Eventually, a total of 585 women conceived, fulfilled trial criteria and provided the primary outcome of gestational glycemia at 28 weeks' gestation, which was assessed by a 75 g three time-point oral glucose tolerance test (OGTT). Those providing primary outcome data were well represented by all three sites (UK:SG:NZ 32%:28%:39%), and comprised predominantly White Caucasian (59%) and Chinese (25%) women. They had the following characteristics: 56% with normal BMI, 63% nulliparous, 66% from top two quintiles of household income [18]. Adherence was good and the intervention did increase plasma micronutrient and myo-inositol concentrations compared with controls when assessed a month after starting supplementation (preconception), with these increments sustained through to at least 28 weeks' gestation [23].

The primary outcome of gestational glycemia was not different between control ($n = 290$) and intervention ($n = 295$) groups; and with adjustment for the randomization factors of site and ethnicity, and other prespecified prognostically important covariates of maternal age, prepregnancy BMI, preconception smoking, parity, family history of diabetes, and baseline glucose at recruitment, none of the group differences in glucose concentrations during the OGTT were statistically significant at the pre-specified $p < 0.017$ which accounts for multiple comparisons [adjusted mean differences in fasting glucose 0.001 (95% confidence interval [CI] –0.06, 0.06) mmol/L; 1 h-glucose 0.29 (–0.02, 0.62) mmol/L; 2 h-glucose 0.26 (0.04, 0.55) mmol/L; these values are the anti-log of the beta coefficients previously published] [18].

NiPPeR Secondary Outcomes

The trial had a number of prespecified secondary outcomes and included below are the ones where analyses have been completed (Table 1). Given that these were not primary outcomes of the trial, with the trial not powered accordingly, the following findings will need confirmation in further studies.

Table 1. Summary of the secondary outcomes of the NiPPeR trial

Outcome	Control	Intervention	Adjusted risk ratio (95% CI)
	Number of cases/ Total (%)	Number of cases/ Total (%)	
Preterm delivery (<37 weeks)	27/292 (9.2%)	17/293 (5.8%)	0.43 (0.22, 0.82)[a]
Late preterm delivery (34^{+0}–36^{+6} weeks)	22/292 (7.5%)	13/293 (4.4%)	0.41 (0.20, 0.85)[a]
Preterm prelabor rupture of membranes (PPROM; <37 weeks)	19/280 (6.8%)	8/277 (2.9%)	0.39 (0.16, 0.97)[a]
Preterm delivery associated with PPROM	17/280 (6.1%)	5/277 (1.8%)	0.21 (0.06, 0.69)[a]
Delay in second stage of labor	55/215 (25.6%)	42/220 (19.1%)	0.68 (0.48, 0.95)[b]
Operative delivery for delay in second stage	41/215 (19.1%)	29/220 (13.2%)	0.61 (0.40, 0.93)[b]
Cesarean section delivery	85/292 (29.1%)	84/293 (28.7%)	0.99 (0.76, 1.28)[a]
Major postpartum hemorrhage (>1,000 mL blood loss)	24/292 (8.2%)	9/294 (3.1%)	0.44 (0.20, 0.94)[a]
Small-for-gestational-age[d] (birth weight <10th centile)	21/292 (7.2%)	24/293 (8.2%)	1.34 (0.79, 2.29)[a]
Large-for-gestational-age[d] (birth weight >90th centile)	22/292 (7.5%)	21/293 (7.2%)	0.94 (0.54, 1.63)[a]
Child obesity at age 2 years (BMI >95th centile)	44/245 [18%]	22/239 [9%]	0.51 (0.31, 0.82)[c]

Data extracted from previous publications [18, 25, 28]. [a]Adjusted for site, ethnicity, maternal age, preconception BMI, household income level, parity, smoking, offspring sex (except for LGA and SGA), and (where data was available) 28 weeks' gestation fasting glucose.
[b]Adjusted for site, ethnicity, maternal age, prepregnancy BMI, household income level, previous cesarean section history, and smoking. Not adjusted for parity and epidural use as second stage diagnosis already accounted for these factors.
[c]Adjusted for site, maternal preconception BMI, parity, maternal smoking, offspring sex, and gestational age at delivery.
[d]By RCPCH 2009 UK-WHO growth charts [29].

Time-to-Conception and Clinical Pregnancy Rate

Overall, among 1,437 women providing data, those taking the intervention supplement had a similar time-to-conception as controls; it took 90.5 and 92.0 days for 20% of women in the intervention and control groups to conceive, respectively, with similar clinical pregnancy (viable intrauterine pregnancy at 6 weeks' gestation) rates at the end of a year after recruitment (adjusted hazard ratio 0.98 [95% CI 0.83, 1.15]) [24]. As with previous studies, our trial population also demonstrated that women with overweight or obesity had a longer time-to-conception compared with the nonoverweight/obese. Analyses stratified by BMI at recruitment suggested that intervention may particularly benefit women with overweight (n = 382); they displayed a shorter time-to-conception with the NiPPeR intervention, shortening it to that which was similar to nonoverweight/obese women (20% conception in intervention vs. control: 84.5 vs. 117 days; adjusted hazard ratio at 1 year 1.47 [1.07, 2.02], p = 0.016) [24]. In contrast, there was suggestion that intervention may have exacerbated subfertility in women with obesity (n = 339; adjusted hazard ratio 0.69 [0.47, 1.00]; p = 0.053), although results need to be interpreted with caution given the wide confidence interval and modest sample size [24].

Preterm Delivery and Preterm Prelabor Rupture of Membranes

The intervention reduced the incidence of preterm delivery (adjusted risk ratio [aRR] 0.43 [0.22, 0.82]), particularly late preterm delivery (34^{+0}–36^{+6} weeks' gestation; aRR 0.41 [0.20, 0.85]) and those associated with preterm prelabor rupture of membranes (aRR 0.21 [0.06, 0.69]) compared with controls [18]. However, there were no overall differences in neonatal complications, or in admissions to the neonatal unit.

Major Postpartum Hemorrhage and Postpartum Blood Loss

The incidence of major postpartum hemorrhage (>1,000 mL blood loss) was lower in the intervention group compared with controls (aRR 0.44 [0.20, 0.94]) [18]. Consistent with this finding, the estimated blood loss at delivery was also 10% lower in the intervention group compared with controls, with an adjusted mean difference of 35 mL (95% CI –70, –3.5; p = 0.047) [25].

Labor Duration and Operative Delivery

While overall there were no group differences in the cesarean section delivery rate and the duration of the first stage of labor, the intervention group had a shorter second stage of labor by 20% (adjusted mean difference –12 min [–22.2, –1.2]; p = 0.029), accompanied by a lower risk of experiencing a delay in the second stage of labor (aRR 0.68 [0.48, 0.95]; $p = 0.026$) and reduced operative delivery (cesarean section and instrumental vaginal deliveries) for delayed second stage (aRR 0.61 [0.40, 0.93]; $p = 0.022$) compared with controls [25].

Breastmilk Composition

Even though mothers stopped taking the supplements at delivery, there was a persistence of the NiPPeR intervention effect in breastmilk composition post-delivery. Over the course of the first 3 months postdelivery, compared to controls, breastmilk from women who took the intervention showed higher concentrations of vitamin D (by 20% [95% CI 8, 33]; $p = 0.001$) [26] and zinc (by 11% [95% CI 1.6, 21]; $p = 0.022$) [27].

Infant Weight Gain and Obesity

Despite the lack of difference between control and intervention groups with respect to birthweight (adjusted mean difference 0.05 [95% CI –0.03, 0.13] kg) and the incidences of small- or large-for-gestational age at birth, the trajectory of infant weight gain over the first 2 years of life was less accelerated in the intervention group compared with controls. The incidence of rapid infant weight gain (>1.34 standard deviation score increase from birth to 2 years; known to be associated with future development of adverse metabolic health) was reduced among infants whose mothers received the intervention supplement compared with controls (aRR 0.55 [95% CI 0.34, 0.88]; $p = 0.014$). In the same vein, the incidence of child obesity (BMI >95th centile) at age 2 years was lower among children of the intervention group (aRR 0.51 [0.31, 0.82]; $p = 0.006$) [28]. Sensitivity analyses excluding preterm cases did not materially alter results. Further follow-up of these children is ongoing to assess the persistence of such effects and to evaluate other child outcomes.

Conclusion

Results from the NiPPeR trial support the idea that maternal nutritional supplementation commencing at preconception has the potential to optimize pregnancy outcomes and offspring health. Potentially, modest improvements in maternal nutrient status may have sizeable impact in shaping the long-term health of individual offspring, building resilience against noncommunicable chronic diseases. Given the huge global challenge in tackling the growing prevalence of child obesity and associated metabolic risk, every potential modifiable contributory factor starting with those in would-be-parents (prior to conception) need to be investigated as a potential target for intervention. It is likely that intervention strategies will need to apply customization and risk stratification for best outcomes. The NiPPeR intervention was tested in high-resource settings and care is needed with extrapolating findings to low-middle income countries. Further work is also required within NiPPeR to identify the key supplement components and mechanisms underlying each of the different effects, and the opportunity window for intervention, so supplementation regimens can be further improved for more optimal outcomes.

Acknowledgments

Thank you to the NiPPeR trial participants and their families for their time and involvement; the study research staff, hospital clinical staff at participating centers, and operational support staff for their contributions; the members of the Independent Data Monitoring and Safety Committee for overseeing the conduct of the trial; and the NiPPeR Study Group as listed below:

Benjamin B. Albert (b.albert@auckland.ac.nz), Shelia J. Barton (S.J.Barton@soton.ac.uk), Aristea Binia (aristea.binia@rdls.nestle.com), Hsin Fang Chang (hsin_fang_chang@nuhs.edu.sg), Yap Seng Chong (yap_seng_chong@nuhs.edu.sg), Paula Costello (pc@mrc.soton.ac.uk), Vanessa Cox (vac@mrc.soton.ac.uk), José G.B. Derraik (j.derraik@auckland.ac.nz), Surabhi Devaraj (surabhi.devaraj@rd.nestle.com), Sarah El-Heis (se@mrc.soton.ac.uk), Soo Min Han (clara.han@auckland.ac.nz), Fang Huang (Fang.Huang1@rd.nestle.com), Mrunalini Jagtap (mrunalini.jagtap1@gmail.com), Timothy Kenealy (t.kenealy@auckland.ac.nz), See Ling Loy (Loy.See.Ling@kkh.com.sg), Jaz Lyons-Reid (j.lyons-reid@auckland.ac.nz), Cathriona R. Monnard (Cathriona.Monnard@rd.nestle.com), Heidi Nield (hn@mrc.soton.ac.uk), J. Manuel Ramos (Manuel.Ramos@rdls.nestle.com), Irma Silva-Zolezzi (Irma.SilvaZolezzi@rdls.nestle.com), Sagar K. Thakkar (Sagar.Thakkar@nestle.com), Elizabeth Tham (elizabeth_tham@nuhs.edu.sg), Philip Titcombe (pt6g13@soton.ac.uk), Mark H. Vickers (m.vickers@auckland.ac.nz), Jui-Tsung Wong (csd3589@yahoo.com), Gladys Woon (gladys_woon@nuhs.edu.sg), Hannah Yong (hannah_yong@sics.a-star.edu.sg), Han Zhang (Zhang_Han@sics.a-star.edu.sg).

Conflict of Interest Statement

Public good funding for trial conduct from the UK Medical Research Council, the Singapore National Research Foundation, National Medical Research Council, the National University of Singapore (NUS), and the Agency of Science, Technology and Research (A*STAR) and Gravida, a New Zealand Government Centre of Research Excellence. Funding for provision of the intervention and control supplements and to cover aspects of the fieldwork for the study was provided by Société des Produits Nestlé S.A. under a Research Agreement with the University of Southampton, Auckland UniServices Ltd., SICS, National University Hospital Singapore PTE Ltd. and NUS.

S.-Y.C. is supported by a Singapore NMRC Clinician Scientist Award (MOH-CSAINV19nov-0002) and is part of an academic consortium that has received grants from Nestlé S.A. K.M.G. is supported by the National Institute for Health Research (NIHR Senior Investigator (NF-SI-0515-10042), NIHR Southampton 1000DaysPlus Global Nutrition Research Group (17/63/154) and NIHR Southampton Biomedical

Research Center (IS-BRC-1215-20004)), British Heart Foundation (RG/15/17/3174), and the European Union (Erasmus+ Programme ImpENSA 598488-EPP-1-2018-1-DE-EPPKA2-CBHE-JP). S.-Y.C., W.S.C., and K.M.G. are coinventors on patent filings by Nestlé S.A. relating to the NiPPeR intervention or its components. S.-Y.C. and K.M.G. have received reimbursement from Nestlé Nutrition Institute (NNI) for speaking at scientific conferences and S.-Y.C. has received honoraria from NNI into institutional research funds.

S.-Y.C. made substantial contributions to the design of the work, and to the acquisition, analyses, and interpretation of data, wrote the initial draft of this paper and agrees to be accountable for all the work. W.S.C. made substantial contributions to the design of the work, and to the acquisition, analyses, and interpretation of data, critically reviewed and approved the final version of this paper, and agrees to be accountable for all the work. K.M.G. made substantial contributions to the conception and design of the work, and to the acquisition, analyses, and interpretation of data, critically reviewed and approved the final version of this paper, and agrees to be accountable for all the work.

References

1 Godfrey KM, Gluckman PD, Hanson MA. Developmental origins of metabolic disease: life course and intergenerational perspectives. Trends Endocrinol Metab. 2010;21(4):199–205. https://doi.org/10.1016/j.tem.2009.12.008

2 HAPO Study Cooperative Research Group, Metzger BE, Lowe LP, Dyer AR, Trimble ER, Chaovarindr U, et al. Hyperglycemia and adverse pregnancy outcomes. N Engl J Med. 2008;358(19):1991–2002. https://doi.org/10.1056/NEJMoa0707943

3 Tam WH, Ma RC, Yang X, Li AM, Ko GT, Kong AP, et al. Glucose intolerance and cardiometabolic risk in adolescents exposed to maternal gestational diabetes: a 15-year follow-up study. Diabetes Care. 2010;33(6):1382–4. https://doi.org/10.2337/dc09-2343

4 Chu LCH, Sugiyama T, Ma RCW. Recent updates and future perspectives on gestational diabetes mellitus: an important public health challenge. J Diabetes Investig. 2021;12(11):1944–7. https://doi.org/10.1111/jdi.13670

5 Suwaydi MA, Wlodek ME, Lai CT, Prosser SA, Geddes DT, Perrella SL. Delayed secretory activation and low milk production in women with gestational diabetes: a case series. BMC Pregnancy Childbirth. 2022;22(1):350. https://doi.org/10.1186/s12884-022-04685-0

6 Yu J, Wu Y, Yao D, Song S, Zhang H, Xu X, et al. The effects of maternal and perinatal factors on human milk lipids composition. J Food Compos Anal. 2023;123:105596. https://doi.org/10.1016/j.jfca.2023.105596

7 Rameez RM, Sadana D, Kaur S, Ahmed T, Patel J, Khan MS, et al. Association of maternal lactation with diabetes and hypertension: a systematic review and meta-analysis. JAMA Netw Open. 2019;2(10):e1913401. https://doi.org/10.1001/jamanetworkopen.2019.13401

8 Robinson SM, Crozier SR, Harvey NC, Barton BD, Law CM, Godfrey KM, et al. Modifiable early-life risk factors for childhood adiposity and overweight: an analysis of their combined impact and potential for prevention. Am J Clin Nutr. 2015;101(2):368–75. https://doi.org/10.3945/ajcn.114.094268

9 Aris IM, Bernard JY, Chen LW, Tint MT, Pang WW, Soh SE, et al. Modifiable risk factors in the first 1000 days for subsequent risk of childhood overweight in an Asian cohort: significance of parental overweight status. Int J Obes (Lond). 2018;42(1):44–51. https://doi.org/10.1038/ijo.2017.178

10 Fleming TP, Watkins AJ, Velazquez MA, Mathers JC, Prentice AM, Stephenson J, et al. Origins of lifetime health around the time of conception: causes and consequences. Lancet (London, England). 2018;391(10132):1842–52. https://doi.org/10.1016/S0140-6736(18)30312-X

11 Raab R, Michel S, Gunther J, Hoffmann J, Stecher L, Hauner H. Associations between lifestyle interventions during pregnancy and childhood weight and growth: a systematic review and meta-analysis. Int J Behav Nutr Phys Act. 2021;18(1):8. https://doi.org/10.1186/s12966-020-01075-7

12 Sukumar N, Adaikalakoteswari A, Venkataraman H, Maheswaran H, Saravanan P. Vitamin B12 status in women of childbearing age in the UK and its relationship with national nutrient intake guidelines: results from two National Diet and Nutrition Surveys. BMJ Open. 2016;6(8):e011247. https://doi.org/10.1136/bmjopen-2016-011247

13 Kobylinska M, Antosik K, Decyk A, Kurowska K. Malnutrition in obesity: is it possible? Obes Facts. 2022;15(1):19–25. https://doi.org/10.1159/000519503

14 Neufingerl N, Eilander A. Nutrient intake and status in adults consuming plant-based diets compared to meat-eaters: a systematic review. Nutrients. 2021; 14(1):29. https://doi.org/10.3390/nu14010029

15 Adams JB, Kirby JK, Sorensen JC, Pollard EL, Audhya T. Evidence based recommendations for an optimal prenatal supplement for women in the US: vitamins and related nutrients. Matern Health Neonatol Perinatol. 2022;8(1):4. https://doi.org/10.1186/s40748-022-00139-9

16 Stephenson J, Heslehurst N, Hall J, Schoenaker D, Hutchinson J, Cade JE, et al. Before the beginning: nutrition and lifestyle in the preconception period and its importance for future health. Lancet (London, England). 2018;391(10132):1830–41. https://doi.org/10.1016/S0140-6736(18)30311-8

17 Godfrey KM, Cutfield W, Chan SY, Baker PN, Chong YS, Ni PSG. Nutritional intervention preconception and during pregnancy to Maintain healthy glucose metabolism and offspring health ("NiPPeR"): study protocol for a randomised controlled trial. Trials. 2017;18(1):131. https://doi.org/10.1186/s13063-017-1875-x

18 Godfrey KM, Barton SJ, El-Heis S, Kenealy T, Nield H, Baker PN, et al. *Myo*-inositol, probiotics, and micronutrient supplementation from preconception for glycemia in pregnancy: NiPPeR international multicenter double-blind randomized controlled trial. Diabetes Care. 2021;44(5):1091–9. https://doi.org/10.2337/dc20-2515

19 Watkins OC, Yong HEJ, Sharma N, Chan SY. A review of the role of inositols in conditions of insulin dysregulation and in uncomplicated and pathological pregnancy. Crit Rev Food Sci Nutr. 2020 62(6):1626–73. https://doi.org/10.1080/10408398.2020.1845604

20 Wei J, Heng W, Gao J. Effects of low glycemic index diets on gestational diabetes mellitus: a meta-analysis of randomized controlled clinical trials. Medicine (Baltimore). 2016;95(22):e3792. https://doi.org/10.1097/MD.0000000000003792

21 Zhang J, Ma S, Wu S, Guo C, Long S, Tan H. Effects of probiotic supplement in pregnant women with gestational diabetes mellitus: a systematic review and meta-analysis of randomized controlled trials. J Diabetes Res. 2019;2019:5364730. https://doi.org/10.1155/2019/5364730

22 Laitinen K, Poussa T, Isolauri E; Nutrition, Allergy, Mucosal Immunology and Intestinal Microbiota Group. Probiotics and dietary counselling contribute to glucose regulation during and after pregnancy: a randomised controlled trial. Br J Nutr. 2009;101(11):1679–87. https://doi.org/10.1017/S0007114508111461

23 Godfrey KM, Titcombe PJ, El-Heis S, Albert BB, Elizabeth TH, Barton SJ, et al. Maternal B-vitamin and vitamin D status before, during and after pregnancy, and the influence of supplementation preconception and during pregnancy: pre-specified secondary analysis of the NiPPeR double-blind randomized controlled trial. PLoS Med. 2023;20(12):e1004260. https://doi.org/10.1371/journal.pmed.1004260

24 Chan SY, Barton SJ, Loy SL, Chang HF, Titcombe P, Wong JT, et al. Time-to-conception and clinical pregnancy rate with a myo-inositol, probiotics, and micronutrient supplement: secondary outcomes of the NiPPeR randomized trial. Fertil Steril. 2023;119(6):1031–42. https://doi.org/10.1016/j.fertnstert.2023.01.047

25 Chan SY, Yong HEJ, Chang HF, Barton SJ, Galani S, Zhang H, et al. Peripartum outcomes after combined myo-inositol, probiotics, and micronutrient supplementation from preconception: the NiPPeR randomized controlled trial. Am J Obstet Gynecol MFM. 2022;4(6):100714. https://doi.org/10.1016/j.ajogmf.2022.100714

26 Han SM, Huang F, Derraik JGB, Vickers MH, Devaraj S, Redeuil K, et al. A nutritional supplement during preconception and pregnancy increases human milk vitamin D but not B-vitamin concentrations. Clin Nutr. 2023;42(12):2443–56. https://doi.org/10.1016/j.clnu.2023.09.009

27 Han SM, Devaraj S, Derraik JGB, Vickers MH, Huang F, Dubascoux S, et al. A nutritional supplement containing zinc during preconception and pregnancy increases human milk zinc concentrations. Front Nutr. 2022;9:1034828. https://doi.org/10.3389/fnut.2022.1034828

28 Lyons-Reid J, Derraik JGB, Kenealy T, Albert BB, Nieves JMR, Monnard CR, et al. Impact of preconception and antenatal supplementation with myo-inositol, probiotics, and micronutrients on offspring BMI and weight gain over the first 2 years. BMC Med. 2024;22(1):39. https://doi.org/10.1186/s12916-024-03246-w

29 Cole TJ, Williams AF, Wright CM; RCPCH Growth Chart Expert Group. Revised birth centiles for weight, length and head circumference in the UK-WHO growth charts. Ann Hum Biol. 2011;38(1):7–11. https://doi.org/10.3109/03014460.2011.544139

Shiao-Yng Chan
Department of Obstetrics and Gynaecology
Yong Loo Lin School of Medicine
National University of Singapore
1E Kent Ridge Road
NUHS Tower Block, Level 12
Singapore, 119228, Singapore
obgchan@nus.edu.sg

Published online: November 15, 2024

Szajewska H, Neu J, Shamir R, Wong G, Prentice AM (eds): Shaping the Future with Nutrition. Nestle Nutr Inst Workshop Ser. Basel, Karger, 2024, vol 100, pp 28–45 (DOI: 10.1159/000540140)

Gut Microbiota Assembly Begins at Birth and Needs to Be Nurtured

Jens Walter

APC Microbiome Ireland, School of Microbiology and Department of Medicine, University College Cork – National University of Ireland, Cork, Ireland

Abstract

Humans maintain symbiotic relationships with complex microbial communities in their intestinal tracts that are paramount to their host's health and development. Given their importance, it is essential for the host to reliably acquire key members of the gut microbiota and assemble communities that provide benefits during important windows of host development. Epidemiological studies over the last 2 decades have convincingly shown that clinical and nutritional factors that disrupt early-life microbiome assembly predispose humans to infections and chronic noncommunicable diseases. These connections emphasize the importance of understanding host-microbiome assembly on a mechanistic level, the time windows that are most important for host-microbe crosstalk, and the clinical and lifestyle factors that shape and disrupt symbiotic interactions to develop therapeutic and nutritional strategies to prevent noncommunicable diseases. In this article, I will provide an evolutionary and ecological perspective on when and how humans acquire their gut microbiome, the factors that shape the assembly process, and how the process can be disrupted. I will discuss the most important time windows for both microbiome assembly and the microbiome's impact on development of the immune system. Finally, I will discuss how evolutionary and ecological principles inform strategies to support and restore the gut microbiome early in life.

Introduction

Humans, just like other mammals, harbor complex and cell-rich microbial communities in their intestinal tracts (the gut microbiota or microbiome), that are metabolically active and influence the host through many intricate mechanisms. This relationship can be considered a co-evolved symbiosis as the contributions made by the microbes (such as acquisition of nutrients, resistance to infections, and cues that aid immune system development) advance host fitness and are large enough to shape the evolution of anatomical, immunological, and metabolic features of mammals, as well as their dietary specializations [1]. Given their importance to many aspects of host development, it is essential for mammals to reliably acquire microbial symbionts and assemble communities that provide benefits.

Epidemiological, physiological, and omics-based studies, complemented by experiments in animals, indicate that a large part of the environmental influence on human health and disease is mediated by the gut microbiota [2]. Clinical, environmental, and nutritional factors that disrupt microbiome assembly early in life are consistently linked to the risk of developing acute pathologies and noncommunicable diseases (NCDs). These connections emphasize the importance of understanding, on a mechanistic level, how gut microbial communities are acquired and assemble, the ecological factors that shape this process, and the implications on host development and health. There is further a need to understand the health consequences that arise from a disruption of this process and when microbiomes become altered and "dysbiotic", and to explore strategies to prevent and redress such aberrations.

Here, I will provide an evolutionary and ecological perspective on the timing and dynamics of early-life microbiome acquisition and assembly and the factors that shape and disrupt the process. I will focus specifically on key members of the early-life microbiota that have co-evolved with humans to perform important functions for both the development of the microbial community and the host. I will then discuss research that determined the importance of "windows of opportunity" for both microbiome assembly and the microbiome's impact on the host's immune system. Finally, I will discuss how evolutionary and ecological principles inform strategies to support and nurture the gut microbiome, specifically to redress misconfigurations. Although non-bacterial components of microbiomes, such as the mycobiome and virome, are increasingly recognized as important contributors, this review will focus on bacteria.

When, How, and from Where Do Infants Acquire Their Gut Microbiomes?

Whether healthy human fetuses and the prenatal intrauterine environment (amniotic fluid, placenta) are colonized by microbial communities has become a heated scientific debate [3]. Over the last 10 years, the application of next-generation sequencing has challenged the previously well-accepted "sterile womb hypothesis", and suggestions have been made that live microbes or even whole microbiomes within intrauterine sites contribute to prenatal fetal immune development [4, 5]. The notion of a fetal microbiome, if proven correct, would have major implications for our understanding of how the immune system develops and the mechanisms by which the microbiome is acquired. These interpretations have, however, been questioned because several concurrent studies point to different sources of contamination as the only source of microbial DNA detected in the intrauterine environment [3].

Such disagreement over a fundamental aspect of early-life human development poses a challenge for scientific progress. I was fortunate to participate in a multidisciplinary group of scientists and clinician-scientists to evaluate the scientific evidence from the perspectives of reproductive biology, microbial ecology, bioinformatics, immunology, clinical microbiology, and gnotobiology, to assess possible mechanisms by which the fetus might interact with microbes [6]. The group concluded that the microbial signals in intrauterine environment are likely the result of contamination during the clinical procedures to obtain placental or fetal samples, or during DNA extraction and DNA sequencing. We further concluded that the existence of live and replicating microbial populations, often composed of opportunistic pathogens according to the sequence analysis, is biologically implausible being incompatible with fundamental concepts of immunology, clinical microbiology, and the derivation of germ-free mammals. These conclusions have since been supported by findings from a re-analysis of fifteen published sequence data sets of placental samples [7] and a microbial analysis of mid-trimester amniotic fluid from 692 pregnancies using culture and PCR [8].

Given that the fetus is sterile in utero, acquisition of the microbiota occurs during and after birth, and different sources have been hypothesized for the colonizers of the infant gut [9] (Table 1). Metagenomics with strain-level resolution is increasingly used to determine the origin of strains detected in infants and the modes of transmission. During vaginal birth, the infant is primarily exposed to the vaginal microbiota, which has been hypothesized as a major source for the infant's microbiota. Accordingly, vaginal

Table 1. Sources of microbes transmitted to infants and their relevance for early-life microbiome assembly

Source	Mode of transmission/ dispersal	Characteristics of habitat and microbes present	Relevance for early-life gut microbiome assembly	Relevance for host development
Foetus and the prenatal intrauterine environment (amniotic fluid and placenta)	Vertical	Sterile in most healthy pregnancies. *Streptococcus agalactiae* (known as Group B *Streptococcus*, or GBS) is detectable in a small subset of placentas and can be transmitted to the infant	None	*Streptococcus agalactiae* causes illness in both newborns and mothers
Mothers' vagina	Vertical	Colonized by dense microbial communities that are, in most women, dominated by specialized species of lactobacilli	Vaginal strains of lactobacilli become detectable in infants' fecal samples but lack adaptations to the gut environment and only form relevant populations in the first few days of life. Strains do not seem to persist. It is unknown to what degree early colonization by lactobacilli influences trajectory of microbiome assembly through priority effects	Extensive literature has established clear effects of lactobacilli on immune functions in animals, e.g., mice, but it is unknown if vaginal microbes impact host development in humans
Breast milk	Vertical	Human breastmilk contains complex communities of microbes, but organisms are from cutaneous or oral habitats and likely originate from the mother's skin or the infant's oral microbiota. Bifidobacteria have been reported to be dominant in breast milk, but such findings are highly inconsistent among studies and not supported by culture-based approaches (pointing to contamination)	Unlikely to impact gut microbiome assembly. The microbes that are commonly detected in breast milk lack adaptations to gut environments and do not form relevant populations in the infant's gut	Unknown, but given that the microbial communities present in breastmilk are highly variable and seem to be allochthonous contaminants, it is unlikely they have an evolved role in infant development
Maternal fecal microbiota	Vertical	Complex microbial communities highly adapted to the gut ecosystem	Highly important as it provides a source of well adapted organisms that arrive early in the infant's life, and thus show elevated persistence and effects on community assembly trajectory through priority effects	Important role in infant development

Table 1 (continued)

Source	Mode of transmission/ dispersal	Characteristics of habitat and microbes present	Relevance for early-life gut microbiome assembly	Relevance for host development
Fecal microbiota of father, siblings, and other humans	Horizontal	Complex microbial communities highly adapted to the gut ecosystem	Important, especially in infants born by c-sections or treated by antibiotics that rely on horizontal transmission of gut microbes, and later in life (e.g., during and after weaning) to mature microbiome to an adult stage	Important role for infant development, especially in infants where vertical transmission is interrupted
Skin microbiota	Vertical and horizontal	Complex microbial communities not adapted to the gut ecosystem	Composes microbiome in c-section born infants early in life, but microbes are outcompeted by gut adapted species within weeks of life	Unknown but might predispose infants to immune mediated pathologies
Pets and other environmental sources	Horizontal	Complex microbial communities not adapted to the gut ecosystem of humans	Little evidence that environmental microbial exposures exert larger effects on gut microbiome assembly	Microbial exposure might impact host development, but effect of gut adapted strains that are vertically transmitted is likely to be larger

Lactobacillaceae species are transmitted to the infant and constitute a larger proportion of the fecal microbiota of vaginally born infants. However, lactobacilli only form significant populations over the first days of life [10]. Human breast milk, supposedly containing more than 700 bacterial species providing a daily dose of more than 800,000 bacteria, has also been hypothesized as a source of gut colonists [11]. However, the bacteria detected in breast milk in most studies are characteristic of cutaneous or oral habitats, such as staphylococci (especially *Staphylococcus epidermidis*) and streptococci. These microbes likely originate from the mother's skin or the infant's oral microbiota and do not form relevant populations in the infant's gut [9, 12]. Some studies have reported high proportions of *Bifidobacterium* species in breast milk that overlap with the infant microbiome. However, these findings are not consistent among studies and not supported by findings using culture-based approaches, and it is important to consider that breast milk is a low biomass sample highly susceptible to cross-contamination during sequencing (the so-called splashome) [6]. Instead, metagenomic strain-tracking demonstrates that a substantial proportion of strains acquired by vaginally-born infants postnatally can be traced back to their mother's fecal microbiota [13, 14], indicative of maternal vertical transmission, with the intestinal rather than the vaginal or milk microbiota being the most important source [10].

Microbiome Assembly as a Process of Ecological Succession

Early life acquisition of microbes in vaginally born infants at term results in a dynamic, sequential de novo assembly process that is characterized by ecological succession [9, 11]. Although the process has often been described as chaotic due to the high temporal and compositional variation, common patterns have been detected [15], and several research groups have described 'successional stages' or "phases" where the microbiome matures across specific community types [9, 11, 16]. Patterns of colonization can be explained by the ability of microbes to become acquired (through transmission or dispersal) and the evolutionary adaptations of the bacterial species that allow them to attain relevant population sizes in gastrointestinal niches.

The very first colonizers (pioneer species) that dominate the early stage are aerobic and facultative anaerobic bacterial species such as *Enterococcus*, *Streptococcus*, *Staphylococcus*, and *Enterobacteriaceae* and oxygen tolerant bacteria such as lactobacilli that benefit from the oxygen that is present in the newborn's gut [10, 17]. The lactobacilli that are initially dominant in vaginally born infants but are then lost, are adapted to the ecological conditions of the vagina but lack essential traits to be successful in the infant gut, such as efficient utilization of human milk oligosaccharides (HMOs). Similarly, the aerobic and facultative anaerobic species that bloom during the first few days are overgrown, once oxygen levels decrease, by an expansion of strictly anaerobic species such as *Bacteroides*, *Parabacteroides*, and especially *Bifidobacterium* of fecal origin in a majority of naturally born infants at term [17]. *Bifidobacteria* can reach a prevalence of >90% [18] and a relative abundance of >50% of the total fecal microbiota in breastfed infants over the first few months [19, 20]. The *Bifidobacterium* species and subspecies that dominate, such as *Bifidobacterium longum* subsp. *infantis, Bifidobacterium longum* subsp. *longum, Bifidobacterium bifidum*, and, with more strain to strain variation, *Bifidobacterium breve*, but also some *Bacteroides* species, express specialized membrane transporters and saccharolytic enzymes that allow them to efficiently utilize HMOs [21]. Some types engage in multi-species cross-feeding that involve sugars cleaved from mucus and HMOs (e.g., fucose and sialic acid) as well as metabolic end products such as 1,2-propanediol, contributing to trophic networks [9, 22].

Over time, and especially after weaning, communities become more complex with the arrival of a diverse set of species, many from the phylum *Bacillota* (previously known as *Firmicutes*). These species comprise most of the diversity of the adult microbiota and become dominant later in life, and sometime between the age of 2 and 4, the child's microbiota becomes compositionally equivalent to that of an adult [9]. Interestingly, the *Bacillota* are almost exclusively spore formers that are efficiently acquired through horizontal transmission [23]. This contrasts with *Bifidobacterium* and *Bacteroides* species that do not form spores and rely on efficient vertical transmission from the mother. Evolutionary theory predicts that vertical transmission of symbionts from a parent to their offspring favors mutualism and provides a mechanism by which the host can select specific lineages that provide benefits [24]. Infant-adapted *Bifidobacterium* species protect against infection and support immune development via secretion of metabolites (e.g., indole-3-lactic acid and aromatic lactic acids) [25, 26] and can, therefore, be considered symbionts of humans that provide important functions during a critical window of human development. Interestingly, bifidobacteria levels at 6 months of age were negatively associated with atopic dermatitis and skin prick testing positivity in an observational study in infants raised during COVID-19-associated social distancing measures (the CORAL study) [27].

What Is the Most Important Time Window for Microbiome Assembly and Its Impact on Host Immune Development?

Neonates born at term are not immunologically naïve but are specifically adapted to cope with abrupt exposure to microbial, dietary, and environmental stimuli. Although there is no direct microbial exposure [6], fetal immune education can be driven through maternal-derived microbial metabolites and molecules that pass the placental filter [28]. After birth, the development of the immune system continues in parallel with the assembly of the microbiomes, and comparisons of germ-free and conventional rodents have established a causal contribution of the microbiome to immune development. Germ-free mice can be efficiently colonized with microbiomes during adulthood, and this "conventionalization" corrects most immune deficits detectable in germ-free animals. However, there is an increased realization that the timing of microbial exposure is important for both microbiome assembly and development of immune phenotypes.

Experiments in gnotobiotic mice that were colonized with four bacterial strains and a seed community in succession at different time points revealed that the early arrival of bacterial strains can improve their ecological success during colonization [29]. In addition, the earlier arrival of the four bacterial strains by a few days produced a measurable difference in the long-term trajectory of microbiome assembly. The findings demonstrate the importance of "priority effects", meaning that timing and order of colonization influence the outcomes of competitive and cooperative interactions between organisms and, thereby the trajectory of community assembly [30]. In follow-up experiments, early colonizers either outcompeted (*Akkermansia muciniphila*) or inhibited (*Bacteroides vulgatus*) strains of the same species that arrived later [31], pointing to inhibitory priority effects through niche pre-emption [30]. However, early colonizers can also support colonization of later arrivals through the creation or modification of niches (facilitative priority effects) [30]. These different types of priority effects have been shown to impact the outcomes of competitive interactions between *Bifidobacterium* species in *in vitro* growth cultures containing HMOs. *B. bifidum* and *B. longum* subsp. *infantis*, two avid HMO consumers, dominate through inhibitory priority effects, while strains of *B. breve* with limited HMO-utilization abilities can benefit from facilitative priority effects through the provision of fucose for cross-feeding [32].

Priority effects provide mechanistic explanations for key characteristics of gut ecosystems [29, 31]. Apart from providing a mechanism for the high degree of colonization resistance of gut microbiomes (established organisms bear fitness advantages over later arrivals), priority effects explain why maternally-derived strains, which are likely to arrive early, are more likely to stably colonize than non-maternal strains [10, 13]. In addition, priority effects offer a mechanism by which arrival order (which is largely stochastic) can create differences in gut microbiota composition, thereby potentially contributing to the large inter-individual variation observed in gut microbiomes. Research on priority effects in gut ecosystems is still in its infancy but they are likely a central and pervasive element in the assembly process with significant implications for microbiome modification and restoration efforts.

Gnotobiotic mice can also be used to characterize the impact of the timing of microbiome exposure on the development of the immune system. For example, my group and collaborators characterized immune cell populations in mice in which the timing of colonization was strictly controlled [33]. Comparisons of conventional mice born to colonized mothers with germ-free mice that were conventionalized at birth (meaning they lacked microbial exposure before birth) showed very few differences in immune cell phenotypes. In contrast, delaying conventionalization to 4 weeks after birth (just after weaning) had much larger effects and resulted in altered phenotypes of seven splenic immune cell populations in adulthood. The work complements a large body of literature that has established that lack of early-life exposure to the microbiome and delays in microbiome assembly can lead to immunological deficits and immune-mediated and metabolic pathologies [34].

Overall, the available research supports the concept of a "window of opportunity" early in the postnatal period, during which the acquisition of microbial symbionts makes important contributions to both microbiome assembly and immune system development, with long-lasting consequences. Although the exact length of this window is still not clear, the concept provides a strong rationale to avoid perturbation of microbiome acquisition during the early period and informs efforts to modulate microbiomes to improve host development and health.

Disruptions of Microbiota Assembly through Clinical and Lifestyle Factors

Modern clinical practices, such as cesarean sections (c-sections) and antibiotics, have reduced maternal and infant mortality to very low numbers in affluent societies. However, both practices disrupt microbiome acquisition and assembly. C-sections disrupt the vertical transmission of gut microbes and show a delay in the colonization of bifidobacteria (1–2 months) and in *Bacteroides* (3–4 months), while bacilli (*Enterococcus*, *Staphylococcus*, and *Streptococcus*) and Enterobacteriaceae are increased [15, 17, 18]. Perinatal antibiotic administration to the mothers during birth and postnatal antibiotic treatment of the infants also have long-lasting effects on bifidobacteria, reducing populations throughout the first year of life [15]. C-sections and antibiotics are often used in combination, and they are likely to contribute to the severe disruptions and aberrant successional patterns of microbiome assembly in preterm infants [35].

Formula feeding also alters early-life microbiota composition, although the effect is less obvious on compositional levels [17]. Relative abundance of bifidobacteria is significantly reduced in formula-fed infants but still high, at around 40% [9, 20]. Some findings are something of a conundrum, as diversity and richness of the fecal microbiota, which is commonly assumed to be associated with health in adults, are reduced in breastfed infants [36]. Perhaps the infant microbiome is different in that host factors exert stringent deterministic forces (e.g., HMOs) to select for a highly specific and thus less diverse microbiota [9]. In agreement with this, HMOs are able to reduce the strength of priority effects between *Bifidobacterium* species and effectively select for *B. longum* subsp. *infantis* regardless of colonization order [37]. Apart from proving an efficient mechanism to select for symbionts, the effects of breast milk on the microbiome have ramifications beyond composition, exerting major metabolic effects, changing the metabolite profile of the microbiome, enhancing fermentation, and reducing the pH through the production of acetic acid [26, 38]. The latter two exert further selection pressures on the microbiota that, despite their beneficial effects on pathogen inhibition, could explain the lower microbiome diversity in breast fed infants.

Generally, detectable differences in microbiome composition induced by birth mode, antibiotics, and formula feeding disappear by the age of 12 months, but as discussed above, early periods of microbial acquisition are important for both microbiome trajectory and host immune development. Thus, even transient differences in the pattern of microbiota succession may have long-term effects on the immunological and metabolic development of the host [39]. In fact, epidemiological research convincingly links c-sections, antibiotics, and formula feeding to an increased risk of NCDs. These factors not only appear to alter microbiota assembly in the exposed infants but also seem to contribute to population-wide differences between industrialized and non-industrialized societies. For example, bifidobacteria are underrepresented in the USA, especially when compared to African cohorts [15], and highly co-evolved types, such as *B. longum* subsp. *infantis*, have lower prevalence in industrialized and affluent societies [26]. The epidemiological links between lifestyle factors that disrupt microbiomes and NCDs provide a potential explanation for the increase of NCDs in industrialized societies and provide a strong rationale for therapeutic and nutritional strategies to modulate and restore microbiome assembly early in life.

How Do Evolutionary and Ecological Principles Inform Strategies to Modulate Gut Microbiomes Early in Life?

As no infant formula is yet able to resemble the physiological effects of human milk, breastfeeding remains the best source of nutrition for both infants and their microbiome. Research on improving infant formulas effect on the microbiome, for example through the addition of prebiotics, is very active, and especially the use of HMOs is clearly in agreement with evolutionary and ecological considerations to improve health [40]. However, neither improved formula nor breast milk are sufficient to redress microbiome perturbations caused by cesarean sections and prenatal antibiotics. Different strategies to restore early life microbiome assembly have been proposed and range from vaginal seeding and fecal microbiota transplantation to more defined microbial-based approaches, such as probiotics [41] (Table 2).

Vaginal seeding involves the exposure of c-section infants directly after birth to vaginal secretions of the mother's vagina. Vaginal seeding has been reported to

Table 2. Microbial-based strategies to modulate and restore microbiomes early in life and the evolutionary and ecological principles that determine outcomes

Strategy	Characteristics of the microbes/microbial communities used	Effects on early-life microbiome assembly	Evolutionary and ecological principles	Health effects, safety considerations, and limitations
Vaginal seeding	Undefined microbial communities present in the mother's vagina	Partially restores the faecal microbiota of c-section infants, but effects are specific to certain bacterial groups (e.g., lactobacilli) and only detectable very early in life	Microbes that inhabit the vagina of humans do lack adaptation to form stable populations in the infant's gut. Gut microbes seem to be largely absent and do not become transmitted. Vaginal microbes can colonize early on in high numbers and might impact microbiome assembly through priority effects, but evidence for this is currently lacking in humans	Unclear if early exposure to vaginal microbes and microbial communities impacts host development and health in humans. Safety concerns have been raised as communities are undefined and might contain pathogens, but risk should not be higher than that of a natural vaginal birth and can potentially be mitigated through pathogen testing
Fecal microbiota transplant (FMT)	Undefined microbial communities prepared from fecal samples, preferentially the mother	Efficiently restores the faecal microbiota in c-section born infants to that seen in infants born through vaginal birth	Restores vertical transmission of the fecal microbiome equivalent to levels observed during a healthy vaginal birth. Introduces well-adapted microbes and communities that can initiate and support gut microbiome assembly	Clinical data on the health effects and prevention of NCDs of early-life FMT treatment are lacking. Safety concerns have been raised as communities are undefined and might contain pathogens, but risk should not be higher than that of a natural vaginal birth and can potentially be mitigated through pathogen testing
Probiotic strains and consortia	Defined microbes or microbial consortia	If infant- and HMO adapted microbes are used, strategies can restore important compositional (e.g., domination of bifidobacteria, reduction of opportunistic pathogens) and functional (low pH, high levels of organic acids, bioactive metabolites) features of the early-life microbiome in breastfed infants	Dependent on strain selection, probiotics can aid in the acquisition of key members of the infant gut microbiome that stably colonize and contribute to microbiome assembly and maturation. By doing this, probiotics can redress some of the adverse effects of c-sections and antibiotic use on microbiome assembly	Clinical benefits of probiotics for Necrotizing Enterocolitis (NEC) are well established, but their use in preterm infants is controversial and there is disagreement among organizations if probiotics should be recommended. Effects of probiotics on other pathologies have been extensively studied, but findings are less consistent. There is a lack of well-designed clinical trials that tested whether probiotics that contain autochthonous strains

Table 2 (continued)

Strategy	Characteristics of the microbes/microbial communities used	Effects on early-life microbiome assembly	Evolutionary and ecological principles	Health effects, safety considerations, and limitations
				can prevent NCDs. Good safety record of bifidobacteria and lactobacilli in infants born at term, and composition of products can be defined and controlled. However, small and standardized set of strains might miss important species and functions present in whole microbiomes
Synbiotics	Combination of probiotic strains or consortia with compounds that serve as growth substrates for the microbes (e.g., prebiotics or HMOs)	Same effects as probiotics, but persistence and functionality of strains can be enhanced, especially in formula fed infants	Both traditional prebiotic and HMOs provide resources and thus a niche opportunity to gut microbes that support their ecological performance. HMOs have likely evolved to support key members of the microbiota, such as bifidobacteria	Synbiotics might be able to enhance the health effects of probiotics, but evidence from well-designed clinical studies is lacking. HMOs are diverse and it will be impossible and expensive to reflect their natural diversity in products. Although clearly bifidogenic, traditional prebiotics differ chemically from HMOs and might therefore not exert the same functions. Good safety record

partially restore the fecal microbiota of C-section infants [42], but opinions on its value and relative risk differ among scientists [43]. Vaginal seeding does not restore a microbiota equivalent to that seen in antibiotic-naïve infants born vaginally [44], primarily restoring vaginal lactobacilli, which, as discussed above, lack relevant adaptations and do not persist in the infant gut in detectable proportions over longer periods. In contrast to vaginal seeding, oral inoculation of C-section infants with maternal feces (maternal fecal microbiota transplant) mimics the natural vertical transmission of fecal microbes and does efficiently restore the microbiome towards that of vaginally born infants [44]. Although fecal microbiota transplantation is, from an ecological perspective, highly efficient, there are safety concerns and regulatory hurdles that prevent it from becoming a feasible standard procedure.

An alternative to the complex undefined approaches described above are live bacterial strains or defined microbial consortia. There is a large body of literature on the use of probiotics in both term and preterm infants using a wide variety of strains and strain combinations [45]. Most of this research was conducted with bacteria that are not infant or even gut-adapted, such as *Lactobacilaceae* and *Bifidobacterium lactis*/*animalis*, which have only small effects (if any) on the gut microbiota. However, what is becoming increasingly clear is that, if infant- and HMO-adapted strains are used, probiotics can restore key aspects of infant gut microbiota composition and function [26]. For example, administration of *B. longum* subsp. *infantis* EVC001 in the first month of life restored Bifidobacteriaceae levels to around 80% relative abundance of the fecal microbiota in breastfed infants, and *B. longum* subsub. *infantis* was detectable at counts to 10.81 $\log_{10}$ cells per gram feces [46] and persisted for up to 1 year [47]. The probiotic treatment resulted in higher concentrations of acetate and lactate, decreased fecal pH, altered metabolic profiles, and lowered levels of Proteobacteria [46, 48], indicating both compositional and functional shifts associated with healthy gut microbiota assembly (see above). Even in extremely premature infants, a probiotic product containing four strains of *Bifidobacterium* species autochthonous to the infant gut and one *Lacticaseibacillus rhamnosus* strain led to stable persistence of the *Bifidobacterium* (but not the *L. rhamnosus* strain) long after administration was ceased [48]. The probiotic also accelerated the transition into a mature, term-like microbiome with higher stability and species interconnectivity, and the abundance of *Bifidobacterium* strains were strong predictors of microbiome maturation. Synbiotics, composed of infant-type bifidobacteria and prebiotics, are also being increasingly explored in formula-fed infants and have shown the potential to change *Bifidobacterium* proportions, fecal pH, lactate production closer to the breastfed reference group [49].

The ecological effects detected in these probiotic trials in infants are substantially larger than those observed in probiotic interventions in adults, likely because colonization resistance is low in infants and both priority effects contribute to strain persistence and microbiome maturation [50]. The probiotic strategies also dampened proinflammatory responses and induced other beneficial immune responses [48, 51]. However, it is still unclear if probiotics can prevent NCDs. Clinical benefits are well established for Necrotizing Enterocolitis (NEC) in preterm infants, where probiotics containing autochthonous *Bifidobacterium* species have shown dramatic reductions in NEC and mortality [52, 53]. Despite great heterogeneity among available studies, large meta-analyses of clinical trials have demonstrated the efficacy of multiple-strain probiotics (most containing infant-adapted bifidobacteria) in reducing NEC and all-cause mortality [52]. The beneficial effects of probiotics on NEC can serve as a paradigm for the value of early-life microbiome restoration in a highly perturbed setting.

Conclusions and Outlook

Our understanding of the transmission of gut microbes and the dynamics of microbiome assembly has grown substantially in recent years. The close proximity of the birth canal to the anus is likely, not coincidental but the result of an evolutionary process that, despite the evolutionary trade-offs (e.g., urinary infections), was driven by the importance of a reliable acquisition of health-promoting microbes and communities during what is likely the most critical window for host development. However, many questions remain, especially as they pertain to the questions of if and how delayed and altered microbiome assembly contributes to pathologies. Answering these questions is complicated by the fact that most NCDs that have implicated the early-life microbiome arise much later in life and are relatively rare, thus requiring large long-term and ideally prospective studies in specific risk groups that are difficult to conduct.

Recent research convincingly demonstrated that evolutionary and ecologically informed procedures can redress microbiome aberrations and replenish keystone species in infants born through c-sections, treated with antibiotics, required formula feeding, or combinations thereof. Given that probiotic products that contain autochthonous *Bifidobacterium* strains are available and safe, such products can be recommended. It should also be noted that restoration efforts are likely to remain imperfect if the infant is not breastfed [41]. The combination of probiotics with synbiotic strategies (e.g., HMOs supplementation) is therefore highly promising but still relatively little explored in clinical studies [54]. One must also consider that the small and standardized set of strains might miss important species and functions, and responses will likely vary between individuals and populations from different geographic location. Although much remains to be done in the design of probiotics for the postnatal period, an advantage of an evolutionary approach would be that strategies are aligned with human biology and should, at least in most cases, be beneficial to most infants independent of where they live.

Although research in animal models is promising, clinical proof in humans that microbiome restoration approaches reduce the risk of NCDs is still essentially missing. This research requires large prospective human trials in specific risk groups. Such research should also consider the long-term risk of these strategies. If we assume that microbial strains and metabolites can prevent NCDs, there might also be cases, even within bacterial species that are normally beneficial, that increase the risk in all or a subset of individuals. Regulatory hurdles are also a significant challenge for effective translation [26], as demonstrated by the warning letters issued by the FDA in October 2023 about probiotic products sold for use in hospitalized preterm infants (despite strong evidence that the risk-benefit ratio is strongly in favor of the use of probiotics). Clearly, the risk is never zero, but the design of microbiome restoration approaches on an evolutionary and ecological basis increases the likelihood of those strategies being safe.

Although the early postnatal period is likely the most important period for the gut microbiome to impact long-term health, the relevant time span is likely broader and might extend into weaning. The CORAL study showed that plant-based foods, which support healthy microbiota (e.g., through dietary fiber) [55], positively impacted microbiota development [27]. Given that metabolites from the maternal microbiota cross the placental barrier into the fetus [6] and a diverse healthy diet maintains a diverse microbiota in women that can then be transmitted to the new-born [11], both the maternal diet during pregnancy and the infant's diet during weaning are likely important to nurture microbiome assembly and long-term health.

Conflict of Interest Statement

J.W. has received honoraria and/or paid consultancy from Novozymes, and ByHeart. J.W. received lecture honoraria and travel reimbursement from Nestlé Nutrition Institute. He is further a co-owner of Synbiotic Health, a developer of Synbiotic products, and owns a patent on the probiotic strain *Limosilactobacillus reuteri* PB-W1.

References

1 Ley RE, Hamady M, Lozupone C, Turnbaugh PJ, Ramey RR, Bircher JS, et al. Evolution of mammals and their gut microbes. Science. 2008;320(5883):1647–51. https://doi.org/10.1126/science.1155725.

2 Fan Y, Pedersen O. Gut microbiota in human metabolic health and disease. Nat Rev Microbiol. 2021;19(1):55–71. https://doi.org/10.1038/s41579-020-0433-9.

3 Perez-Munoz ME, Arrieta MC, Ramer-Tait AE, Walter J. A critical assessment of the "sterile womb" and "in utero colonization" hypotheses: implications for research on the pioneer infant microbiome. Microbiome. 2017;5(1):48. https://doi.org/10.1186/s40168-017-0268-4.

4 Mishra A, Lai GC, Yao LJ, Aung TT, Shental N, Rotter-Maskowitz A, et al. Microbial exposure during early human development primes fetal immune cells. Cell. 2021;184(13):3394–409.e20. https://doi.org/10.1016/j.cell.2021.04.039.

5 Rackaityte E, Halkias J, Fukui EM, Mendoza VF, Hayzelden C, Crawford ED, et al. Viable bacterial colonization is highly limited in the human intestine in utero. Nat Med. 2020;26(4):599–607. https://doi.org/10.1038/s41591-020-0761-3.

6 Kennedy KM, de Goffau MC, Perez-Munoz ME, Arrieta MC, Backhed F, Bork P, et al. Questioning the fetal microbiome illustrates pitfalls of low-biomass microbial studies. Nature. 2023;613(7945):639–49. https://doi.org/10.1038/s41586-022-05546-8.

7 Panzer JJ, Romero R, Greenberg JM, Winters AD, Galaz J, Gomez-Lopez N, et al. Is there a placental microbiota? A critical review and re-analysis of published placental microbiota datasets. BMC Microbiol. 2023;23(1):76. https://doi.org/10.1186/s12866-023-02764-6.

8 Romero R, Gervasi MT, DiGiulio DB, Jung E, Suksai M, Miranda J, et al. Are bacteria, fungi, and archaea present in the midtrimester amniotic fluid? J Perinat Med. 2023;51(7):886–90. https://doi.org/10.1515/jpm-2022-0604.

9 Tannock GW. Building robust assemblages of bacteria in the human gut in early life. Appl Environ Microbiol. 2021;87(22):e0144921. https://doi.org/10.1128/AEM.01449-21.

10 Podlesny D, Fricke WF. Strain inheritance and neonatal gut microbiota development: a meta-analysis. Int J Med Microbiol. 2021;311(3):151483. https://doi.org/10.1016/j.ijmm.2021.151483.
11 Linehan K, Dempsey EM, Ryan CA, Ross RP, Stanton C. First encounters of the microbial kind: perinatal factors direct infant gut microbiome establishment. Microbiome Res Rep. 2022;1(2):10. https://doi.org/10.20517/mrr.2021.09.
12 Moossavi S, Sepehri S, Robertson B, Bode L, Goruk S, Field CJ, et al. Composition and variation of the human milk microbiota are influenced by maternal and early-life factors. Cell Host Microbe. 2019;25(2):324–35.e4. https://doi.org/10.1016/j.chom.2019.01.011.
13 Ferretti P, Pasolli E, Tett A, Asnicar F, Gorfer V, Fedi S, et al. Mother-to-infant microbial transmission from different body sites shapes the developing infant gut microbiome. Cell Host Microbe. 2018;24(1):133–45.e5. https://doi.org/10.1016/j.chom.2018.06.005.
14 Mitchell CM, Mazzoni C, Hogstrom L, Bryant A, Bergerat A, Cher A, et al. Delivery mode affects stability of early infant gut microbiota. Cell Rep Med. 2020;1(9):100156. https://doi.org/10.1016/j.xcrm.2020.100156.
15 Korpela K, de Vos WM. Early life colonization of the human gut: microbes matter everywhere. Curr Opin Microbiol. 2018;44:70–8. https://doi.org/10.1016/j.mib.2018.06.003.
16 Beller L, Deboutte W, Falony G, Vieira-Silva S, Tito RY, Valles-Colomer M, et al. Successional stages in infant gut microbiota maturation. mBio. 2021;12(6):e0185721. https://doi.org/10.1128/mBio.01857-21.
17 Shao Y, Forster SC, Tsaliki E, Vervier K, Strang A, Simpson N, et al. Stunted microbiota and opportunistic pathogen colonization in caesarean-section birth. Nature. 2019;574(7776):117–21. https://doi.org/10.1038/s41586-019-1560-1.
18 Martin R, Makino H, Cetinyurek Yavuz A, Ben-Amor K, Roelofs M, Ishikawa E, et al. Early-life events, including mode of delivery and type of feeding, siblings and gender, shape the developing gut microbiota. PLoS One. 2016;11(6):e0158498. https://doi.org/10.1371/journal.pone.0158498.
19 Cho S, Samuel TM, Li T, Howell BR, Baluyot K, Hazlett HC, et al. Interactions between *Bifidobacterium* and *Bacteroides* and human milk oligosaccharides and their associations with infant cognition. Front Nutr. 2023;10:1216327. https://doi.org/10.3389/fnut.2023.1216327.
20 Harmsen HJ, Wildeboer-Veloo AC, Raangs GC, Wagendorp AA, Klijn N, Bindels JG, et al. Analysis of intestinal flora development in breast-fed and formula-fed infants by using molecular identification and detection methods. J Pediatr Gastroenterol Nutr. 2000;30(1):61–7. https://doi.org/10.1097/00005176-200001000-00019.
21 Marcobal A, Sonnenburg JL. Human milk oligosaccharide consumption by intestinal microbiota. Clin Microbiol Infect. 2012;18 suppl 4(0 4):12–5. https://doi.org/10.1111/j.1469-0691.2012.03863.x.
22 Cheng CC, Duar RM, Lin X, Perez-Munoz ME, Tollenaar S, Oh JH, et al. Ecological importance of cross-feeding of the intermediate metabolite 1,2-propanediol between bacterial gut symbionts. Appl Environ Microbiol. 2020;86(11):e00190-20. https://doi.org/10.1128/AEM.00190-20.
23 Browne HP, Neville BA, Forster SC, Lawley TD. Transmission of the gut microbiota: spreading of health. Nat Rev Microbiol. 2017;15(9):531–43. https://doi.org/10.1038/nrmicro.2017.50.
24 Fisher RM, Henry LM, Cornwallis CK, Kiers ET, West SA. The evolution of host-symbiont dependence. Nat Commun. 2017;8:15973. https://doi.org/10.1038/ncomms15973.
25 Laursen MF, Sakanaka M, von Burg N, Morbe U, Andersen D, Moll JM, et al. Bifidobacterium species associated with breastfeeding produce aromatic lactic acids in the infant gut. Nat Microbiol. 2021;6(11):1367–82. https://doi.org/10.1038/s41564-021-00970-4.
26 Mills DA, German JB, Lebrilla CB, Underwood MA. Translating neonatal microbiome science into commercial innovation: metabolism of human milk oligosaccharides as a basis for probiotic efficacy in breast-fed infants. Gut Microb. 2023;15(1):2192458. https://doi.org/10.1080/19490976.2023.2192458.
27 Korpela K, Hurley S, Ford SA, Franklin R, Byrne S, Lunjani N, et al. Association between gut microbiota development and allergy in infants born during pandemic-related social distancing restrictions. Allergy. 2024;79(7):1938–51. https://doi.org/10.1111/all.16069.
28 Gomez de Aguero M, Ganal-Vonarburg SC, Fuhrer T, Rupp S, Uchimura Y, Li H, et al. The maternal microbiota drives early postnatal innate immune development. Science. 2016;351(6279):1296–302. https://doi.org/10.1126/science.aad2571.
29 Martinez I, Maldonado-Gomez MX, Gomes-Neto JC, Kittana H, Ding H, Schmaltz R, et al. Experimental evaluation of the importance of colonization history in early-life gut microbiota assembly. Elife. 2018;7:e36521. https://doi.org/10.7554/eLife.36521.
30 Fukami T. Historical contingency in community assembly: integrating niches, species pools, and priority effects. Annu Rev Ecol Evol Syst. 2015;46(1):1–23. https://doi.org/10.1146/annurev-ecolsys-110411-160340.
31 Segura Munoz RR, Mantz S, Martinez I, Li F, Schmaltz RJ, Pudlo NA, et al. Experimental

evaluation of ecological principles to understand and modulate the outcome of bacterial strain competition in gut microbiomes. ISME J. 2022;16(6):1594–604. https://doi.org/10.1038/s41396-022-01208-9.
32 Ojima MN, Jiang L, Arzamasov AA, Yoshida K, Odamaki T, Xiao J, et al. Priority effects shape the structure of infant-type Bifidobacterium communities on human milk oligosaccharides. ISME J. 2022;16(9):2265–79. https://doi.org/10.1038/s41396-022-01270-3.
33 Archer D, Perez-Munoz ME, Tollenaar S, Veniamin S, Cheng CC, Richard C, et al. The importance of the timing of microbial signals for perinatal immune system development. Microbiome Res Rep. 2023;2(2):11. https://doi.org/10.20517/mrr.2023.03.
34 Gensollen T, Iyer SS, Kasper DL, Blumberg RS. How colonization by microbiota in early life shapes the immune system. Science. 2016;352(6285):539–44. https://doi.org/10.1126/science.aad9378.
35 Mercer EM, Arrieta MC. Probiotics to improve the gut microbiome in premature infants: are we there yet? Gut Microb. 2023;15(1):2201160. https://doi.org/10.1080/19490976.2023.2201160.
36 Yelverton CA, Killeen SL, Feehily C, Moore RL, Callaghan SL, Geraghty AA, et al. Maternal breastfeeding is associated with offspring microbiome diversity; a secondary analysis of the MicrobeMom randomized control trial. Front Microbiol. 2023;14:1154114. https://doi.org/10.3389/fmicb.2023.1154114.
37 Laursen MF, Roager HM. Human milk oligosaccharides modify the strength of priority effects in the Bifidobacterium community assembly during infancy. ISME J. 2023;17(12):2452–7. https://doi.org/10.1038/s41396-023-01525-7.
38 Martin FP, Tytgat HLP, Krogh Pedersen H, Moine D, Eklund AC, Berger B, et al. Host-microbial co-metabolites modulated by human milk oligosaccharides relate to reduced risk of respiratory tract infections. Front Nutr. 2022;9:935711. https://doi.org/10.3389/fnut.2022.935711.
39 Dogra SK, Kwong Chung C, Wang D, Sakwinska O, Colombo Mottaz S, Sprenger N. Nurturing the early life gut microbiome and immune maturation for long term health. Microorganisms. 2021;9(10):2110. https://doi.org/10.3390/microorganisms9102110.
40 Berger B, Porta N, Foata F, Grathwohl D, Delley M, Moine D, et al. Linking human milk oligosaccharides, infant fecal community types, and later risk to require antibiotics. mBio. 2020;11(2):e03196-19. https://doi.org/10.1128/mBio.03196-19.
41 Korpela K, de Vos WM. Infant gut microbiota restoration: state of the art. Gut Microb. 2022;14(1):2118811. https://doi.org/10.1080/19490976.2022.2118811.
42 Dominguez-Bello MG, De Jesus-Laboy KM, Shen N, Cox LM, Amir A, Gonzalez A, et al. Partial restoration of the microbiota of cesarean-born infants via vaginal microbial transfer. Nat Med. 2016;22(3):250–3. https://doi.org/10.1038/nm.4039.
43 van Best N, Dominguez-Bello MG, Hornef MW, Jasarevic E, Korpela K, Lawley TD. Should we modulate the neonatal microbiome and what should be the goal? Microbiome. 2022;10(1):74. https://doi.org/10.1186/s40168-022-01281-4.
44 Korpela K, Helve O, Kolho KL, Saisto T, Skogberg K, Dikareva E, et al. Maternal fecal microbiota transplantation in cesarean-born infants rapidly restores normal gut microbial development: a proof-of-concept study. Cell. 2020;183(2):324–34.e5. https://doi.org/10.1016/j.cell.2020.08.047.
45 Depoorter L, Vandenplas Y. Probiotics in pediatrics. A review and practical guide. Nutrients. 2021;13(7):2176. https://doi.org/10.3390/nu13072176.
46 Frese SA, Hutton AA, Contreras LN, Shaw CA, Palumbo MC, Casaburi G, et al. Persistence of supplemented *Bifidobacterium longum* subsp. *infantis* EVC001 in breastfed infants. mSphere. 2017;2(6):e00501-17. https://doi.org/10.1128/mSphere.00501-17.
47 O'Brien CE, Meier AK, Cernioglo K, Mitchell RD, Casaburi G, Frese SA, et al. Early probiotic supplementation with B. infantis in breastfed infants leads to persistent colonization at 1 year. Pediatr Res. 2022;91(3):627–36. https://doi.org/10.1038/s41390-020-01350-0.
48 Samara J, Moossavi S, Alshaikh B, Ortega VA, Pettersen VK, Ferdous T, et al. Supplementation with a probiotic mixture accelerates gut microbiome maturation and reduces intestinal inflammation in extremely preterm infants. Cell Host Microbe. 2022;30(5):696–711.e5. https://doi.org/10.1016/j.chom.2022.04.005.
49 Phavichitr N, Wang S, Chomto S, Tantibhaedhyangkul R, Kakourou A, Intarakhao S, et al. Impact of synbiotics on gut microbiota during early life: a randomized, double-blind study. Sci Rep. 2021;11(1):3534. https://doi.org/10.1038/s41598-021-83009-2.
50 Walter J, Maldonado-Gomez MX, Martinez I. To engraft or not to engraft: an ecological framework for gut microbiome modulation with live microbes. Curr Opin Biotechnol. 2018;49:129–39. https://doi.org/10.1016/j.copbio.2017.08.008.
51 Henrick BM, Rodriguez L, Lakshmikanth T, Pou C, Henckel E, Arzoomand A, et al.

Bifidobacteria-mediated immune system imprinting early in life. Cell. 2021;184(15):3884–98.e11. https://doi.org/10.1016/j.cell.2021.05.030.

52 Bui A, Johnson E, Epshteyn M, Schumann C, Schwendeman C. Utilization of a high potency probiotic product for prevention of necrotizing enterocolitis in preterm infants at a level IV NICU. J Pediatr Pharmacol Ther. 2023;28(5):473–5. https://doi.org/10.5863/1551-6776-28.5.473.

53 Tobias J, Olyaei A, Laraway B, Jordan BK, Dickinson SL, Golzarri-Arroyo L, et al. Bifidobacteriumlongum subsp. infantis EVC001 administration is associated with a significant reduction in the incidence of necrotizing enterocolitis in very low birth weight infants. J Pediatr. 2022;244:64–71.e2. https://doi.org/10.1016/j.jpeds.2021.12.070.

54 Button JE, Autran CA, Reens AL, Cosetta CM, Smriga S, Ericson M, et al. Dosing a synbiotic of human milk oligosaccharides and B. infantis leads to reversible engraftment in healthy adult microbiomes without antibiotics. Cell Host Microbe. 2022;30(5):712–25.e7. https://doi.org/10.1016/j.chom.2022.04.001.

55 Armet AM, Deehan EC, O'Sullivan AF, Mota JF, Field CJ, Prado CM, et al. Rethinking healthy eating in light of the gut microbiome. Cell Host Microbe. 2022;30(6):764–85. https://doi.org/10.1016/j.chom.2022.04.016.

Jens Walter
APC Microbiome Ireland
School of Microbiology and Department of Medicine
4.05 Biosciences Building
University College Cork – National University of Ireland
Cork, T12 YT20, Ireland
jenswalter@ucc.ie.

Published online: November 15, 2024

Szajewska H, Neu J, Shamir R, Wong G, Prentice AM (eds): Shaping the Future with Nutrition. Nestle Nutr Inst Workshop Ser. Basel, Karger, 2024, vol 100, pp 46–55 (DOI: 10.1159/000540135)

Understanding the Ovarian Clock – Essential Knowledge for Pediatricians

Zhongwei Huang[a, b, c]

[a]Department of Obstetrics and Gynaecology, National University Hospital, Singapore, Singapore; [b]NUS Bia Echo Asia Centre for Reproductive Longevity and Equality, Yong Loo Lin School of Medicine, National University of Singapore, Singapore, Singapore; [c]Departments of Obstetrics and Gynaecology & Physiology, Yong Loo Lin School of Medicine, National University of Singapore, Singapore, Singapore

Abstract

A woman is born with her life-time supply of eggs, and these are surrounded by a group of cells, the follicular cells, which form the ovarian follicles. The ovarian follicles will determine a woman's entire reproductive lifespan (presence of menstrual cycles and length of fertility) and healthspan (i.e., quality of life). The ovarian follicles are at their peak numbers in utero and start to decline upon birth. This decline continues nonlinearly throughout the girls' growth to adolescence and in adulthood. This decline also represents the inevitable loss of fertility, culminating in women's menopause, where the ovaries have too few ovarian follicles left to result in monthly menstrual bleeding. The role of these ovarian follicles is vital for a woman's fertility as they safeguard the eggs within them. Importantly, the hormones secreted by the ovarian follicles (e.g., estradiol) maintain a woman's healthspan by ensuring optimal cardiovascular, musculoskeletal, and neurocognitive health. Conditions that accelerate the loss of these ovarian follicles or shorten the already limited ovarian lifespan will result in systemic issues detrimental to women's health. Yet, the biological processes that determine the ovarian clock remain understudied and this phenomenon needs attention to ensure that novel diagnostics and therapeutics are discovered for optimal women's reproductive health.

Introduction

A Girl Is Born with a Finite Number of Eggs

Every baby girl is born with her life-time supply of eggs. These eggs are surrounded by a layer of follicular cells which nurture their growth and development. The flattened layer of follicular cells surrounding the egg is known as the primordial follicles [1], which form the true ovarian reserve a girl will ever possess in her lifetime. In women, all primordial follicles are formed in the fetus between 6- and 9-months' gestation. During this period, a marked loss of oocytes occurs due to apoptosis until approximately 1–2 million ovarian follicles are left at birth. The number of primordial follicles decreases progressively because of their recruitment during ovarian folliculogenesis for ovulation [2], until about 1,000 follicles or less [3], at which point ovulation culminates as menopause, which usually occurs at ~50 years of age (see Fig. 1). The decline in number of ovarian follicles is not linear throughout a girl's lifetime, with optimal fertility occurring around the age of 18–31 years. This then follows a steep decline in the number of ovarian follicles from age 37 years and beyond leading to a reduction in fertility.

The primordial follicles will remain quiescent in early life and are activated at the time of puberty, where the "Central clock," the hypothalamic–pituitary–ovarian (HPO) axis, matures and results in increased pulsatile release of gonadotropin-releasing hormone (GnRH) from the hypothalamus to the pituitary gland. This is likely due to polygenic influence, with epigenetic

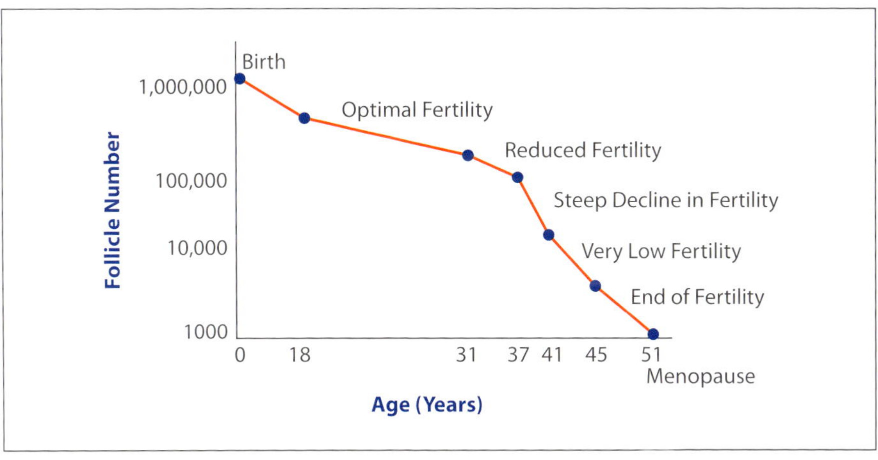

Fig. 1. A girl's ovarian lifespan is dependent on the number of ovarian follicles she is born with, and it is a downwards trajectory until the clinical menopause as the girl goes into adolescence and adulthood.

mechanisms providing coordination and transcriptional plasticity to the genetic network governing the onset of puberty [4]. With the onset of puberty, ovarian folliculogenesis commences under the influence of follicle-stimulating hormone (FSH) and luteinizing hormone (LH), resulting in the secretion of high levels of estrogens (e.g., estradiol) in a positive feedback loop. The elevated levels of estrogens will kick-start the physical changes seen during puberty, including thelarche and adrenarche. Further, the uterus will respond to the cyclical production of estrogens and result in menarche, which is the first presentation of menstrual bleeding due to the shedding of the endometrium from withdrawal of estrogen [5]. The first ovulation usually takes place approximately 6–9 months after menarche due to an initially immature positive feedback mechanism of estrogen [5].

The Central Clock and the Ovarian Clock

The onset of puberty in girls is controlled by GnRH neurons. The development of this pulsatile gonadotropin secretion ultimately triggers the first ovulation, giving rise to the potential for reproduction [6]. The now matured "Central Clock" is able to generate the pulses necessary to initiate ovarian folliculogenesis cyclically, thereby allowing the ovaries to recruit from their finite pool of primordial follicles monthly for selection of one dominant follicle for ovulation. The onset of the Central Clock will work in concert with the ovarian clock to regulate ovarian folliculogenesis. However, dysregulation of ovarian folliculogenesis will result in ovulatory disorders [7]. This also marks the continual loss of ovarian follicles throughout a woman's life, and the rate of decline is dependent on each phase of her adult life as depicted in Figure 1.

The Ovary Dictates a Girl's Reproductive Lifespan and Healthspan

The ovarian clock begins ticking from birth, and continual loss of ovarian follicles results in the inevitable end of reproductive lifespan. The ovarian follicles contain oocytes for fertility and reproduction. The granulosa cells growing in these follicles are vital in nurturing the developing oocytes during ovarian folliculogenesis. Their production of estrogens is pivotal for a woman's healthspan. Estrogen is essential in sustaining both bone and cardiovascular health. It protects bones by inactivating osteoclast activity, preventing osteoporosis in both estrogen-deficient and postmenopausal women [8]. Furthermore, estrogen affects plasma lipids by increasing high-density lipoproteins and triglyceride levels while decreasing low-density lipoproteins and total plasma cholesterol. Consequentially, this aids in the reduction in the risk of coronary artery disease by creating a healthy lipid profile which is cardio-protective [9].

Concept of Reproductive Ageing in Women

The ovary is one of the first organs to functionally decline with age, which results in an overt decline of general health, especially afflicting the neurocognitive, cardio-metabolic, musculoskeletal, and reproductive systems [10]. This biological phenomenon occurs way before other bodily systems [11], resulting in increased morbidity and all-cause mortality in women who suffers from early menopause less than 40 years of age. The timing of menopause is critically implicated with later menopause being associated with greater life expectancy and reduced all-cause mortality [12]. Furthermore, if menopause occurs before age 40 years, in a condition known as premature ovarian insufficiency (POI), these women are at increased risk of osteoporosis, cardiovascular, and neurologic diseases, leading to increased risks of premature death [13]. An interesting phenomenon observed in pregnant mothers with female fetuses demonstrated that in utero events such as low birth weight and diethylstilbestrol exposure could result in the female fetus being at risk of early natural menopause in the future [14]. This exemplifies the importance of protecting a girl from unnecessary exposure or risks that may adversely affect her future reproductive lifespan and healthspan. This can be achieved through careful considerations of the diet and environment from in utero life to birth and beyond.

Impact of Health Sequelae from Early Initiation of Puberty and Early Menarche

Many epidemiological studies have demonstrated that rising childhood levels of obesity and ponderosity are associated with earlier menarche in girls [15]. Early-life and childhood nutrition are likely to exert a significant impact on the timing of puberty onset [16]. Nutritional status is considered one of the most important factors involved in pubertal development whereas much as 25% of the variation in the timing of puberty may be attributable to nutritional causes [17]. Furthermore, the long-term adverse health consequences such as increased risks of breast cancer, obesity, diabetes mellitus, cardiovascular diseases, and lower bone mineralization can collectively heighten mortality risk [16]. Additionally, a history of either early or late menarche was associated with a higher risk for adverse cardiovascular outcomes (e.g., coronary arterial disease later in life) [18]. Therefore, utmost attention should be paid to modifiable risk factors (e.g., diet, obesity, life-style factors) that influence age of menarche as a potential means to mitigate life-time risks of chronic diseases that reduce lifespan and healthspan.

The Irreversibility of the Human Ovarian Clock

The human ovarian clock undergoes an irreversible loss of ovarian follicles and this ovarian ageing is attributable to multiple biological processes at play. The local microenvironment of the ovarian follicle in the ovary directly influences the quality of the eggs in the ovary [19] and subsequent fertility in women. The tissue and cellular components in the ovary, stroma, immune cells, granulosa cells, mitochondria, and extracellular matrix, undergo intrinsic changes during the ageing process. These are influenced by oxidative stress and inflammation. Genetic factors, telomerase activity, epigenetics, and nutritional factors can accelerate the ovarian ageing process [20]. Lamentably, ovarian and reproductive ageing remains an understudied area. However, attempts to maintain the quality and quantity of follicles in animal models through manipulating the aging pathways can hold promising potential to prolong female reproductive lifespan and healthspan. Understanding the molecular events driving ovarian aging and menopause and the interventional strategies to offset these events will open doors to discover ways to enhance true healthy longevity for women [21], beginning from birth to childhood. Novel methods to increase the primordial follicle pool during the preconception period need to be further investigated to exploit this window of opportunity.

Approach to "Ovarian Clock" – What the Pediatrician Should Know

A common presentation to the pediatrician is the irregular menstruation once an adolescent reaches menarche. Adolescent girls who have not reached menarche within 5 years after thelarche and amenorrhoeic girls without secondary sexual characteristics development by the age of 13 (2 SD above the mean age of 11) should also undergo evaluation [22]. The American College of Obstetricians and Gynecologists defined irregular menstrual cycles in the first-year post menarche as normal due to the immature hypothalamic–pituitary–ovarian axis. However, further evaluation of irregular menstrual cycles may be warranted if the following features are noted: (1) between 1 and 3 years postmenarche with menstrual cycles <21 days OR >45 days (2) more than 3 years postmenarche with menstrual cycles <21 days OR >35 days OR <8 cycles/year (3) more than 1-year postmenarche with menstrual cycles >90 days for any one cycle (4) primary amenorrhea by age 15 or >3 years postthelarche [23].

Amenorrhea is characterized by the complete absence or cessation of menses. The occurrence of amenorrhea before and after menarche defines primary and secondary amenorrhea, respectively [24]. Careful medical evaluation and management should be warranted for these women with amenorrhea. Additionally, the presence or absence of secondary sexual characteristics can offer more insights to the causes of amenorrhea. Causes of amenorrhea include anatomical or functional anomalies of the genital tract, hormonal disorders such as hyperprolactinemia, and hypogonadotrophic hypogonadism, including rare genetic syndromes. The girl's reproductive hormonal profile such as FSH, LH, thyroid-stimulating hormone (TSH), prolactin, and androgen levels should be assessed. It is vital to determine the cause of irregular menstrual cycles and ensure that the cycles return to prevent the short- and long-term sequelae of estrogen imbalance. It poses an increased risk for cardiometabolic diseases, osteoporosis, premature menopause, and endometrial cancer, curtailing one's healthspan.

The most common causes of irregular cycles and amenorrhea are hypothalamic amenorrhea, polycystic ovarian syndrome (PCOS), and POI (see Fig. 2).

POI and PCOS represent the extreme ends of the ovarian lifespan spectrum, with POI associated with a decreased lifespan and PCOS to an increased lifespan. However, these ovarian-specific conditions can result in serious consequences to a girl's future reproductive health and general well-being.

Premature Ovarian Insufficiency – Ovaries Which Aged Prematurely

POI results from a premature depletion of the ovarian pool of primordial follicles or in certain genetic conditions such as X-chromosome–related genetic disorders (e.g., Turner's syndrome). This is diagnosed clinically based on serum FSH and estradiol levels, measured on at least two separate occasions with an interval of more than 4 weeks, with a continuously elevated FSH levels (greater than 25 IU/L) [25]. Concurrently, the serum level of anti-Mullerian hormone (AMH), a marker for ovarian reserve in routine clinical use, may become abnormally low for her age. This is a debilitating condition afflicting 1% of the women before age 40 years globally. A significant proportion of women with POI die from cardiovascular diseases. Furthermore, POI is among the main factors associated with premature mortality, following diabetes and arterial hypertension [26], leading to premature mortality. Compounding the issue, women with POI experience increased odds of developing individual chronic conditions and multimorbidities such as diabetes, hypertension, heart disease, stroke, arthritis, osteoporosis, depression, and anxiety [27]. Although it

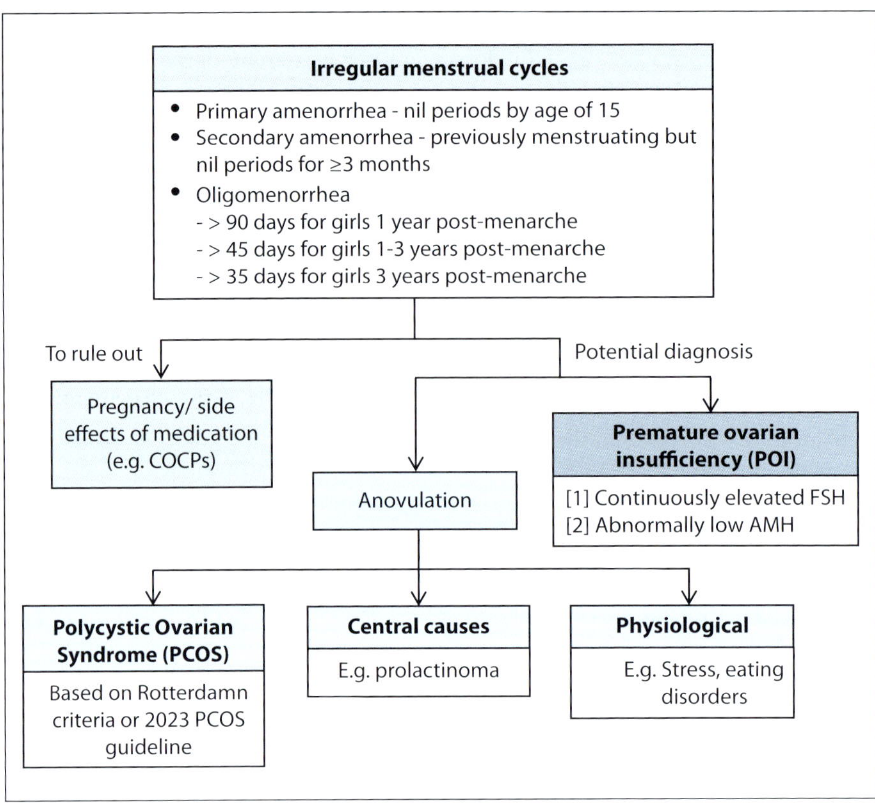

Fig. 2. Diagnostic approach to irregular menstrual cycles.

is crucial to determine the cause of POI, the identification of possible causative genes and selection of candidate genes for POI confirmation remains to be elucidated [28]. Nonetheless, diagnosing POI is essential for pediatricians to ensure early referral for subspecialist and multidisciplinary care. This will allow the girl or adolescent suffering from POI to receive timely and appropriate management such as hormonal replacement therapy and nutritional and lifestyle advice for optimal health.

PCOS – The Ovary with Increased Lifespan

PCOS is one of the most common endocrine disorders in women of reproductive age with a prevalence of up to 20%. Their clinical presentation includes irregular menstrual cycles, hirsutism, also known as excessive hair growth, and subfertility [29]. Importantly, PCOS is associated with metabolic disorders such as insulin resistance, impaired glucose tolerance, type 2 diabetes mellitus, dyslipidemia, and cardiovascular risk factors [30]. Ironically, women with PCOS were observed to experience delayed ovarian ageing, as reflected by the slower rate of decline in serum concentrations of AMH over time [31]. Furthermore, genetic susceptibility to later onset of menopause is associated with higher PCOS risk—which suggests a common mechanism that retards ovarian ageing. Interestingly, PCOS-susceptibility alleles are associated with higher serum AMH concentrations in women. While the very low level of AMH in POI women reflects low numbers of primordial follicles, the higher AMH level in PCOS women suggest a higher number of primordial follicles. High AMH level consequently inhibits the recruitment of further primordial follicles, possibly representing more efficient use of the primordial ovarian pool [32]. Therefore, accurate diagnosis of PCOS in a girl or adolescent will be pivotal to guide appropriate nutrition and lifestyle modifications to mitigate the aforementioned risks for obesity, diabetes, and cardiovascular disorders.

Conclusion

The ovarian clock needs to be emphasized to the pediatricians as it has far-reaching reproductive and health implications to a growing girl. Conditions that affect the ovarian lifespan, such as POI and PCOS, must be identified to enlist preventive measures to maintain good health and well-being. Understanding that there will be an irrevocable and inevitable loss of ovarian follicles from birth, girls must have appropriate and sufficient nutrition to build up their bodily reserves (e.g., peak bone mass, muscular development) as well as adequate lifestyle modifications like aerobic exercise to ensure optimal healthspan.

Acknowledgement

I would like to acknowledge Miss Jovin Lee for formatting and technical assistance.

Conflict of Interest Statement

The author has no conflicts of interest to declare.

Funding Sources

Z.H. is partially funded by the NUS Bia Echo Asia Centre for Reproductive Longevity and Equality. Z.H. received lecture honoraria and travel reimbursement from Nestlé Nutrition Institute.

Author Contributions

Z.H. conceived, researched, and wrote the manuscript.

References

1 Huang Z, Wells D. The human oocyte and cumulus cells relationship: new insights from the cumulus cell transcriptome. Mol Hum Reprod. 2010;16(10): 715–25. https://doi.org/10.1093/molehr/gaq031.

2 Baker TG. Radiosensitivity of mammalian oocytes with particular reference to the human female. Am J Obstet Gynecol. 1971;110(5):746–61. https://doi.org/10.1016/0002-9378(71)90271-7.

3 Faddy MJ, Gosden RG, Gougeon A, Richardson SJ, Nelson JF. Accelerated disappearance of ovarian follicles in mid-life: implications for forecasting menopause. Hum Reprod. 1992;7(10):1342–6. https://doi.org/10.1093/oxfordjournals.humrep.a137570.

4 Ojeda SR, Lomniczi A, Sandau U, Matagne V. New concepts on the control of the onset of puberty. Endocr Dev. 2010;17:44–51. https://doi.org/10.1159/000262527.

5 Rosenfield RL, Lipton RB, Drum ML. Thelarche, pubarche, and menarche attainment in children with normal and elevated body mass index. Pediatrics. 2009;123(1):84–8. https://doi.org/10.1542/peds.2008-0146.

6 Herbison AE. Control of puberty onset and fertility by gonadotropin-releasing hormone neurons. Nat Rev Endocrinol. 2016;12(8):452–66. https://doi.org/10.1038/nrendo.2016.70.

7 Urman B, Yakin K. Ovulatory disorders and infertility. J Reprod Med. 2006;51(4):267–82.

8 Klein-Nulend J, van Oers RF, Bakker AD, Bacabac RG. Bone cell mechanosensitivity, estrogen deficiency, and osteoporosis. J Biomech. 2015;48(5): 855–65. https://doi.org/10.1016/j.jbiomech.2014.12.007.

9 Hong MK, Romm PA, Reagan K, Green CE, Rackley CE. Effects of estrogen replacement therapy on serum lipid values and angiographically defined coronary artery disease in postmenopausal women. Am J Cardiol. 1992;69(3): 176–8. https://doi.org/10.1016/0002-9149(92)91300-s.

10 Recognizing the importance of ovarian aging research. Nat Aging. 2022;2(12):1071–1072. https://doi.org/10.1038/s43587-022-00339-0.

11 Khan SS, Singer BD, Vaughan DE. Molecular and physiological manifestations and measurement of aging in humans. Aging Cell. 2017;16(4):624–33. https://doi.org/10.1111/acel.12601.

12 Gold EB. The timing of the age at which natural menopause occurs. Obstet Gynecol Clin North Am. 2011;38(3):425–40. https://doi.org/10.1016/j.ogc.2011.05.002.

13 Lokkegaard E, Jovanovic Z, Heitmann BL, Keiding N, Ottesen B, Pedersen AT. The association between early menopause and risk of ischaemic heart disease: influence of hormone therapy. Maturitas. 2006;53(2):226–33. https://doi.org/10.1016/j.maturitas.2005.04.009.

14 Langton CR, Whitcomb BW, Purdue-Smithe AC, Sievert LL, Hankinson SE, Manson JE, et al. Association of in utero exposures with risk of early natural menopause. Am J Epidemiol. 2022;191(5): 775–86. https://doi.org/10.1093/aje/kwab301.

15 Biro FM, Khoury P, Morrison JA. Influence of obesity on timing of puberty. Int J Androl. 2006; 29(1):272–90. https://doi.org/10.1111/j.1365-2605.2005.00602.x.

16 Calcaterra V, Verduci E, Magenes VC, Pascuzzi MC, Rossi V, Sangiorgio A, et al. The role of pediatric nutrition as a modifiable risk factor for precocious puberty. Life (Basel). 2021;11(12):1353. https://doi.org/10.3390/life11121353.

17 Soliman A, De Sanctis V, Elalaily R. Nutrition and pubertal development. Indian J Endocrinol Metab. 2014;18(suppl 1):S39–47. https://doi.org/10.4103/2230-8210.145073.

18 Lee JJ, Cook-Wiens G, Johnson BD, Braunstein GD, Berga SL, Stanczyk FZ, et al. Age at menarche and risk of cardiovascular disease outcomes: findings from the national heart lung and blood institute-sponsored women's ischemia syndrome evaluation. J Am Heart Assoc. 2019;8(12):e012406. https://doi.org/10.1161/JAHA.119.012406.

19 Babayev E, Duncan FE. Age-associated changes in cumulus cells and follicular fluid: the local oocyte microenvironment as a determinant of gamete quality. Biol Reprod. 2022;106(2):351–65. https://doi.org/10.1093/biolre/ioab241.

20 Camaioni A, Ucci MA, Campagnolo L, De Felici M, Klinger FG; Italian Society of Embryology Reproduction and Research SIERR. The process of ovarian aging: it is not just about oocytes and granulosa cells. J Assist Reprod Genet. 2022;39(4): 783–92. https://doi.org/10.1007/s10815-022-02478-0.

21 Dong L, Teh DBL, Kennedy BK, Huang Z. Unraveling female reproductive senescence to enhance healthy longevity. Cell Res. 2023;33(1): 11–29. https://doi.org/10.1038/s41422-022-00718-7.

22 The Practice Committee of the American Society for Reproductive Medicine. Current evaluation of amenorrhea. Fertil Steril. 2008;90(suppl 3):219–25. https://doi.org/10.1016/j.fertnstert.2008.08.038.
23 ACOG Committee Opinion No. 651: Menstruation in girls and adolescents—using the menstrual cycle as a vital sign. Obstet Gynecol. 2015;126:e143–6. https://doi.org/10.1097/AOG.0000000000001215.
24 Deligeoroglou E, Athanasopoulos N, Tsimaris P, Dimopoulos KD, Vrachnis N, Creatsas G. Evaluation and management of adolescent amenorrhea. Ann N Y Acad Sci. 2010;1205:23–32. https://doi.org/10.1111/j.1749-6632.2010.05669.x.
25 Wesevich V, Kellen AN, Pal L. Recent advances in understanding primary ovarian insufficiency. F1000Res. 2020;9:F1000 Faculty Rev-1101. https://doi.org/10.12688/f1000research.26423.1.
26 Blümel JE, Mezones-Holguín E, Chedraui P, Soto-Becerra P, Arteaga E, Vallejo MS. Is premature ovarian insufficiency associated with mortality? A three-decade follow-up cohort. Maturitas. 2022;163: 82–7. https://doi.org/10.1016/j.maturitas.2022.06.002.
27 Xu X, Jones M, Mishra GD. Age at natural menopause and development of chronic conditions and multimorbidity: results from an Australian prospective cohort. Hum Reprod. 2020;35(1):203–11. https://doi.org/10.1093/humrep/dez259.
28 Chon SJ, Umair Z, Yoon MS. Premature ovarian insufficiency: past, present, and future. Front Cell Dev Biol. 2021;9:672890. https://doi.org/10.3389/fcell.2021.672890.
29 Louwers YV, Laven JSE. Characteristics of polycystic ovary syndrome throughout life. Ther Adv Reprod Health. 2020;14:2633494120911038. https://doi.org/10.1177/2633494120911038.
30 Teede HJ, Misso ML, Costello MF, Dokras A, Laven J, Moran L, et al. Recommendations from the international evidence-based guideline for the assessment and management of polycystic ovary syndrome. Hum Reprod. 2018;33(9):1602–18. https://doi.org/10.1093/humrep/dey256.
31 Mulders AG, Laven JS, Eijkemans MJ, de Jong FH, Themmen AP, Fauser BC. Changes in anti-Müllerian hormone serum concentrations over time suggest delayed ovarian ageing in normogonadotrophic anovulatory infertility. Hum Reprod. 2004;19(9):2036–42. https://doi.org/10.1093/humrep/deh373.
32 Day FR, Hinds DA, Tung JY, Stolk L, Styrkarsdottir U, Saxena R, et al. Causal mechanisms and balancing selection inferred from genetic associations with polycystic ovary syndrome. Nat Commun. 2015;6:8464. https://doi.org/10.1038/ncomms9464.

Zhongwei Huang
Department of Obstetrics and Gynaecology
National University of Singapore
NUHS Tower Block, Level 12, 1E Kent Ridge Road
Singapore, 119228, Singapore
obgzwh@nus.edu.sg

Published online: November 15, 2024

Szajewska H, Neu J, Shamir R, Wong G, Prentice AM (eds): Shaping the Future with Nutrition. Nestle Nutr Inst Workshop Ser. Basel, Karger, 2024, vol 100, pp 56–70 (DOI: 10.1159/000540139)

Human Milk Research, More to Learn?

Norbert Sprenger[a] Cathriona R. Monnard[b]

[a]Gastrointestinal Health, Nestlé Institute of Health Sciences, Lausanne, Switzerland; [b]Metabolic Health, Nestlé Institute of Health Sciences, Lausanne, Switzerland

Abstract

Human milk is the recommended sole source of nutrition for infants during the first 6 months of age, thanks to its composition rich in nutritious and bioactive components. Progress in analytics has allowed for a detailed description of its components and their variability within and among mothers. This is especially valid for the human milk oligosaccharides (HMOs) that represent one of the major human milk compound groups. The stages of lactation and maternal genotypes are the main contributors to the variability of HMOs, although other maternal and environmental factors also contribute to the variation, which may be important for adaptation in evolutionary terms. Today, mainly individual HMOs or structural groups of HMOs were associated with infant outcome measures, ranging from anthropometry to immunity and brain development (social and cognitive skills). Mechanistic insights can partly explain some findings, yet there is a lack of consistency between the different observational studies of breastfed infants. Gaining a better understanding of the reasons behind these disparate findings is the key element going forward. Furthermore, studying human milk components, like HMOs, and their expected benefits using a systems biology approach can reveal further important insights. Here, we discuss recent findings with the perspective to learn more about the link to health outcomes.

Introduction

Milk production is a unique characteristic of mammals, including diverse species from egg-laying mammals, like echidnas and the platypus, to humans. Sharing a common ancestry and evolutionary adaptation are important hallmarks to consider when investigating the biology of milk and lactation. We may paraphrase this based on a classic statement as "nothing in milk makes sense except in the light of evolution" [1].

The common ancestry of mammals goes back over 200 million years to the so-called synapsids or proto-mammals. These laid eggs with shells intolerant to desiccation, which depended on glandular skin secretions for moisture and antimicrobial properties. These skin secretions are thought to have evolved into a component-rich secretion seen today as milk in mammals [2]. It is noteworthy that milk is thought to have evolved from a secretion rich in protective or bioactive components to the one we see today that is rich in both nutritive and bioactive components.

The study of human milk biology made great strides with the advancement of analytics. A primary focus is on the composition of individual components, aimed in an engineer-like manner to understand the biology at a molecular level, component by component. Today, a shift from such a molecular approach to a more integrative organismal or systems biology approach is needed to fully appreciate milk and its role in infant development [3].

An epidemiology-based approach looking, overall, for differences between breastfed and nonbreastfed infants is an important basis that considers milk holistically. This approach, together with the study of breastfeeding promotion [4] and a randomized trial design of preterm infant feeding with donor human milk or cows' milk-based formula [5], established the importance of human milk feeding for early postnatal development and long-term health.

Hence, the WHO and UNICEF recommend exclusive, on-demand breastfeeding for the first 6 months. From the age of 6 months, children should begin eating safe and adequate complementary foods while continuing to be breastfed for up to 2 years and beyond [4]. Generally, breastfeeding allows for the age-appropriate growth of infants during the first 6 months, although an adequate nutritional status of the mother is the key to this end. Among the benefits for infants, reduced risks for infection-related morbidity, dental caries, and malocclusions are generally reported, together with benefits for brain development and reduction of overweight and diabetes later in life [5].

In this context, some key questions include what factors affect human milk composition, how does variation in the composition affect infant development, and how do different milk components interact with each other and influence infant development? Herein, we discuss these aspects, zooming in on one bioactive milk component group, the human milk oligosaccharides (HMOs).

Variation in Milk Composition: Adaptation to Infant Needs?

The human milk composition varies, and variation is an important feature in biology and evolution for adaptation. We can differentiate intra- and interindividual variation. For the former, milk compositional change over the time of lactation is probably the best described example. Most of the reported milk components change over the course of lactation from colostrum (first 4–5 days), transitional milk (5–14 days), to mature (above 10–14 days), and late milk (>90 days). Given the change in volume intake over time as the infant grows, the actual intake of some specific components may remain rather constant. Another example is diurnal variation with a significant circadian variation reported in a recent systematic review for tryptophan, fats, triacylglycerol, cholesterol, iron, melatonin, cortisol, and cortisone over the day [6]. Such variations may play a role in the child's growth and development and be adapted to nutritional and chronobiological needs. Last, but not least, differences in the composition of fore- and hindmilk, particularly with respect to fat concentration, have been proposed to play an important role in self-control during feeding, with potential implications for weight gain and growth [7].

Variation in the milk composition between mothers may be due to many factors, such as genetics, the physiological and nutritional status of the mother, and her habitual diet, which seems to have a key impact, particularly for fatty acid intake [8]. Diets rich in sea food, for example, are associated with a higher content of docosahexaenoic acid and arachidonic acid in human milk [9].

Variation of Oligosaccharides in Human Milk

Just like many other components in human milk, individual HMO concentrations and HMO profiles also vary. To understand how the variation is brought about, we need to first understand how HMOs are made. The canonical pathway of HMO synthesis starts with lactose. Lactase synthase, a heterodimer of alpha-lactalbumin and the soluble variant of beta-1,4-galactosyltransferase 1, catalyzes the assembly of lactose from UDP-galactose and glucose. Elongation of lactose to the different HMOs occurs via the stepwise addition of further monosaccharides (i.e., galactose, *N*-acetylglucosamine, *N*-acetylgalactosamine, fucose, and sialic acid) in different directions by specific glycosyltransferases as recently reviewed [10].

Among the involved glycosyltransferases, the fucosyltransferases FUT2 and FUT3 lead to a pronounced variation in HMO composition. Humans are polymorphic for both FUT2 and FUT3, defining the phenotypical secretor and Lewis types, respectively. In mothers, this genetic variability translates in their milk to a lack or variability of FUT2-dependent HMOs (e.g., 2′-fucosyllactose (2′-FL), lacto-*N*-fucopentaose I (LNFP-I)), or FUT3-dependent HMOs (e.g., LNFP-II and 3-fucosyllactose (3-FL)). Due to the polymorphism in FUT2 and FUT3 activities, four distinct milk groups can be distinguished (Fig. 1a) [11]. Additional variability is also linked to the maternal blood groups A and AB. Mothers with these blood groups, who also express a functional FUT2 enzyme, synthesize a so-called A-tetrasaccharide in milk, which is composed of trisaccharide 2′-FL with an additional alpha-linked *N*-acetylgalactosamine [12].

Due to substrate use and availability during the presence or absence of FUT2 and FUT3, other HMOs that are not directly made by those enzymes can also be affected. This is due to different donor and acceptor substrate availabilities for HMO synthesis. The examples include 3-FL and LNFP-III, with 3-FL being higher throughout lactation and LNFP-III being slightly higher in transitional milk when FUT2 is missing. Other sialylated HMOs, like 3′-sialyllactose (3′-SL) and sialyllacto-*N*-tetraose c (LST-c), are not affected by the FUT2 and -3 polymorphism (Fig. 1a).

Next to genetic polymorphism, the time of lactation is a second important parameter affecting the HMO composition and profiles. Most HMO concentrations decrease over time. Only a few, especially 3-FL, and to some extent 3′-SL, increase in concentration over the course of lactation. In milk from mothers giving birth at term or preterm, this pattern of decreasing and increasing HMO concentrations as lactation progresses looks very similar [13]. Hence, the program of HMO synthesis regulation appears to start with the establishment of lactation, independent of the infant's gestational age. Yet, few statistically significant differences of specific sialylated HMOs were observed between the milk of mothers following term or preterm birth with the HMOs 3′-SL, LST-b, and DSLNT higher and 6′-SL and LST-c lower in the milk of mothers who gave birth to preterm infants. To what extent these changes reflect the different maternal physiological state or an adaptation to the preterm infant's need is not known. In evolutionary terms, it is unlikely to reflect adaptation, as it is only thanks to recent medical advances that preterm infants survive beyond birth.

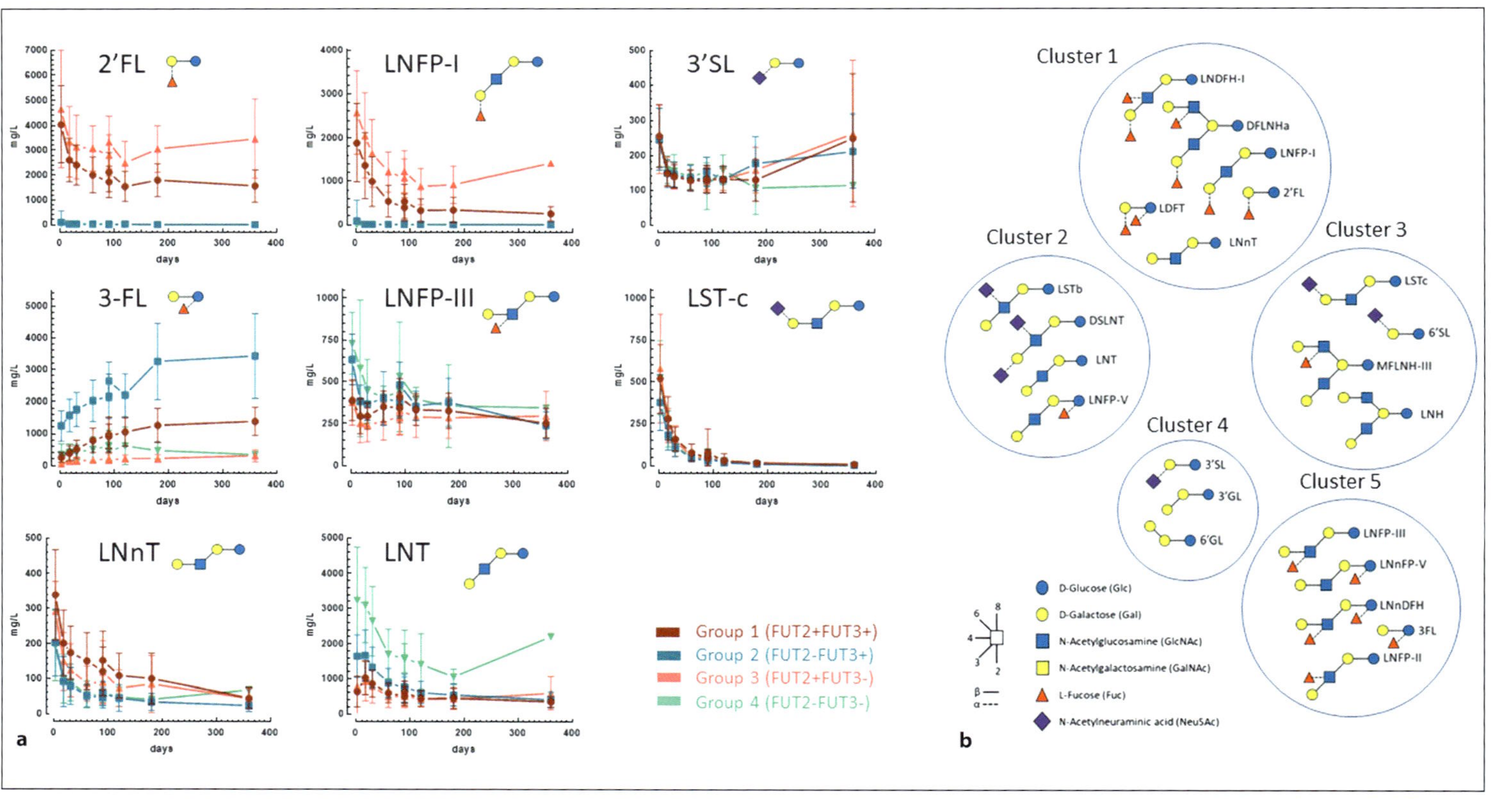

Fig. 1. a Individual HMOs, representative of different HMO clusters, are plotted by the milk group over the time of lactation. Graphs are redrawn from published data [11, 12]. **b** Summary of HMO clusters identified in Lefebvre et al., 2020 [12], also seen similarly in independent unpublished data (Fabio Mainardi, personal communication). Means with standard deviation are shown. The legend shows the monosaccharides and the type and direction of linkages between them, forming the different HMOs shown.

The mode of delivery, parity, and prepregnancy body mass index are other factors that have been associated with the HMO composition in maternal milk [11]. Generally, the observed differences are small and their physiological significance for infant development is questionable.

Among extrinsic factors that may affect the HMO composition, the environment and season at birth may somewhat affect the HMO composition [14, 15]. Both may be due to changes in the maternal diet. Concerning maternal nutritional status, little is known, in part due to the challenges associated with dietary intake assessment and the lack of standardized milk collection and HMO analyses. Although some studies report no association between maternal nutrition and HMO concentrations in mature human milk [16], others have reported negative associations between unmetabolized folic acid from supplementation and concentrations of total HMOs and 3′-sialyllactose [17], indicating that modifiable factors, such as a maternal diet, have the potential to impact HMO concentrations.

Human Milk, the Gut Microbiome, and Infant Development

Postnatal early life development is intimately linked with the colonization and development of the gut microbiota. Numerous studies underscore the link between different microbial groups and healthy infant development [18]. In short, increasingly, attention is focused on the importance of age-appropriate gut microbiota development, appreciating not only the role of specific microbes and microbial communities, but especially the importance of having the right microbes and microbial communities at the right time during early development.

At birth, the infant's gut starts to be colonized, first by more oxygen-tolerant bacteria, followed by more oxygen-sensitive bacterial groups, like bifidobacteria. These generally represent the most prominent group during the exclusive breastfeeding period. With the introduction of animal milk-based formula milk, and especially once weaning food is introduced around 6 months of age, the gut microbiota starts to diversify [19]. The development of the gut microbiota can be elegantly summarized and described using infant-age discriminant bacterial taxa or their functional capacity selected through specific algorithms [19]. A reference microbiota development profile can be established using longitudinal microbiota data from vaginal born, 4–6-month-old exclusively breastfed and normally growing infants, not exposed to antibiotics. Once such a reference microbiota is established, we can compare it to the microbiota development seen in partially breastfed or formula-fed infants, or even to those exposed to antibiotic treatment. Notably, microbiota development in early life is affected by early life nutrition [19]. Undigested milk components from formula or human milk primarily nourish the gut microbiota and HMOs as first fibers are certainly the major component to this end.

With the aforementioned information in mind, research into human milk, especially HMO benefits, will need to integrate the impact of human milk on the gut microbiota. For example, associations between individual HMOs and health conditions or developmental outcomes may look rather different in the presence or absence of specific bifidobacteria that can metabolize (or not) the specific HMOs (Fig. 2). Olm et al. recently reported on the infant microbiota, including bifidobacteria in industrialized and nonindustrialized populations [21]. Industrialized populations were characterized by a lower prevalence of HMO utilization-related gene clusters and more diverse *Bifidobacterium* species than that of infants from nonindustrialized geographies, who had a higher abundance of *B. infantis*, a *Bifidobacterium* species highly adapted to HMO utilization.

Infant Development and Human Milk Oligosaccharides

Infant Growth

Age-appropriate growth is a key indicator of child development and health. Nutrition is one of the key drivers of growth alterations due to under- or overnutrition, which may bear long-term health consequences. The gut microbiota helps to extract nutrients and energy from undigested food. Hence, it is

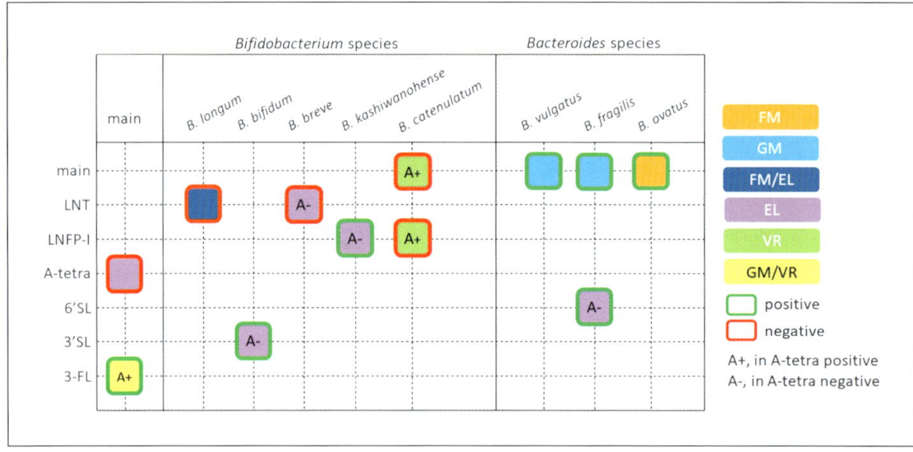

Fig. 2. Associations to brain development outcome measures with HMOs or *Bifidobacterium* and *Bacteroides* species alone (main effects) and with interactions between HMOs and *Bifidobacterium* and *Bacteroides* species. The figure is redrawn from [20]. EL, expressive language; FM, fine motor; GM, gross motor; VR, visual receptive.

plausible that HMOs, likely through their modulation of the gut microbiota, may impact infant growth parameters. Today, many studies have investigated whether HMOs are associated with growth in breastfed infants. Table 1 highlights the observations gathered so far.

Most studies investigated term-born normally-growing infants, where several HMOs were identified as being linked to specific infant growth measures. Despite this, there is generally little consistency among the different studies. The reasons are manifold and range from different study designs to differences in the period of growth assessment, to differences in the gut microbiota, a variable generally not integrated into the analysis. Notably, the reported associations are generally of a small effect size and within the normal range considered as healthy growth.

Among the more consistently observed associations are specific sialylated HMOs, primarily 3′-SL, which showed positive associations with length and weight measures. Interestingly, in two independent cohorts of Malawian mother–infant dyads, the sum of sialylated HMOs was reported to be higher in the milk of mothers nursing normally growing infants than the concentration in the milk of mothers whose infants showed stunted growth [24]. Basic research modeling, a possible mechanism of

Table 1. Associations reported for HMOs and different growth measures

Growth indicator/status	Infant age (months)	Associated HMOs	
		Positive	Negative
Normal versus stunted growth		Fucosyl-HMOs Sialyl-HMOs	
Length	6 to 12	HMO abundance	
	5	LNFP-I + III and DFLNHa	
	3 to 12	2′-FL	LNnT and LST-b
	5	3′-SL and LDFT	LNnT and DFLNH
	6	2′-FL and LNnDFH	3-FL and MFLNH-III
	12	Fucosyl-HMOs	6′-SL, LNnT, and neutral nonfucosylated HMOs
Weight	6		LNFP-I
	1 to 6		LNFP-II
	3 to 12	2′-FL and 3-FL	LNnT
	0 to 5	2′-FL	LNnT
	2 to 6	3′-SL and 6′-SL	
	5	3′-SL	LST-c
	0 to 4	3′-SL and LST-c	
Head circumference	3 to 12	FUT2 negative milk	
	6	LDFT and LNDFH-I	MFLNH-III
Weight, length, and head circumference	0 to 4	No association seen in secretor-positive versus secretor-negative milk	

Summarized based on findings from [10, 22, 23].

action, was later elaborated. The data suggest that sialylated oligosaccharides (primarily 3′-SL), isolated from bovine milk, modulate bone remodeling [25]. The identified pathway involves the gut microbiota and specific gut-epithelial sensor cells, called tuft cells that trigger immune mediators, which direct bone remodeling activity. In a pig model, however, a recent study did not identify any difference in growth in early life by supplementing a milk replacer with 3′-SL or not [26].

Infant Infections

Since the early days of HMO benefit research, it has become clear that one of the key reasons why human milk is so rich in its diversity and abundance of HMOs is to provide protection from infections. This is primarily related to the fact that HMOs are not digested and represent structures, such as those covering the luminal gut surface in the form of mucous and glycocalyx that are the first pathogen anchor points. Additionally, HMOs drive gut microbiota development, which is an important part of the layered defense system in the gut. Mechanistically, several HMOs were shown to bind specific viral and bacterial pathogens. In some cases, this was shown to partly block adhesion to host cells. In other cases, HMOs were also shown to interfere with bacterial pathogen cell-wall synthesis, making them more fragile to antibiotics, for example. Additionally, specific HMOs may dampen inflammation, a mechanism proposed to alter some bacterial pathogens that induce a proinflammatory environment to outcompete commensal bacteria and settle in the gut [10].

In breastfed infants, several HMOs, and among them, mainly alpha-1,2 fucosylated HMOs that depend on a functional FUT2 enzyme, were associated with protection from infectious diarrhea and morbidity (Table 2). Yet, LNFP-II, the main

Table 2. Associations reported for HMOs and immunity-related outcomes

Measure	Infant age (months)	HMOs
Necrotizing enterocolitis	Preterm	DSLNT
	Preterm	HMO diversity
IgE-eczema	48	2′-FL and FUT2-positive milk
Cow milk protein allergy	18	LNFP-III, LNFP-I, 6′-SL, and DSLNT
Sensitization	12	HMO profile a
Diarrhea	9	2′-Fucosyl-HMOs
	9	2′-FL
	ca 11	2′-Fucosyl-HMOs
Morbidity	3	LNFP-II
	4	2′-Fucosyl-HMOs
Respiratory infections	0–6	FUT2-positive milk (including 2′-Fucosyl-HMOs)

Summarized based on findings from [10, 27].

FUT3-dependent HMO, was also associated with lower morbidity. Hence, redundancy among some HMOs and structure-function specificity among others may exist. Another factor to consider is the infant genotype. It is well-established that depending on the pathogen, FUT2 positive (secretor) or FUT2 negative (nonsecretor) genotypes are more or less susceptible [28]. Consequently, the infant genotype may confound associations related to infections. In a mother–infant cohort from Bangladesh that had no milk collection, maternal FUT2 and -3 genotypes, as a proxy for the HMO profiles and other milk glycans, and infant FUT2 and -3 genotypes were determined. The assessment of infection risks by maternal or infant genotype only showed reduced risks for infant respiratory infections during the first 6 months of age when infants were breastfed by FUT2-positive mothers [27]. This indicates that breast milk containing alpha-1,2-fucosylated glycans (including HMOs) may provide some protection independent of the infant FUT2 genotype. Notably, infants in this cohort generally showed a high abundance of *B. infantis*, well-equipped with enzymes to metabolize HMOs, which may partly explain the findings.

Infant Allergies

Sensitization and manifestation of allergies is a major concern and indicator of inappropriate immune competence development. In a systematic review, early life microbiota development was observed as being the most critical for allergic sensitization, such as for eczema or asthma, driven most consistently by a greater relative abundance of *Bacteroidaceae*, *Clostridiaceae*, and *Enterobacteriaceae* and a lower relative abundance of *Bifidobacteriaceae* and *Lactobacillaceae* [29]. In a cohort of breastfed infants with a hereditary risk for allergies, infants born via C-section showed a delay in establishing a bifidobacterial-dominated microbiota at 3 months of age, especially when they received breast milk deficient in FUT2-dependent HMOs [30]. These infants appeared to manifest an earlier onset of IgE-mediated allergies, like eczema, at 2 years of age [31]. Despite the exploratory nature and weakness of the identified association, it seems worthwhile to further explore the role of the early microbiome development in combination with HMOs for immune competence development as recently reviewed [18].

In other studies, individual HMOs, like LNFP-III, -I, 6′-SL, and DSLNT, were associated with cows' milk protein allergy [32] and HMO profiles for sensitization [33]. In an animal model of allergic diarrhea, 6′-SL and 2′-FL were shown to alleviate symptoms through a mast cell stabilizing mechanism. Mechanistically, DSLNT may help to reduce mast-cell chymase, a serine protease, activity that is causally linked to gut epithelial damage and inflammation [34], while LNFP-III and -I represent Lewis X and H1 epitopes, respectively. Both may interact with dendritic cells via the receptor DC-SIGN.

Infant Cognitive and Social Emotional Development

Today, several fucosylated and sialylated HMOs in human milk were reportedly associated with different infant cognitive outcome measures (Table 3). Some of these oligosaccharides, namely, 3′-SL and 6′-SL, are also found in mouse milk, allowing their study in physiological conditions using mutant mice dams deficient in 3′-SL or 6′-SL, cross-feeding wild-type pups. Such experimental models allowed to further corroborate the role of both 3′-SL and 6′-SL in cognitive development [43]. Little is known mechanistically, yet several mechanisms have been proposed, including effects via the gut microbiome or their role as a conditionally essential nutrient supporting brain development. Isotope labeling and gene expression studies in rodents indicate that sialic acid from milk (largely in the form of 3′-SL and 6′-SL) is catabolized [44]. Yet, this may trigger endogenous synthesis needed for rapid brain growth and development. In humans, a recent study observed an association between 6′-SL and social skill development mediated by myelination, a mechanism strongly dependent on sialic acid bound to gangliosides [35]. The same study found associations between 3-FL and other fucosylated HMOs and language development that were not mediated by myelination.

Since different HMOs may act through specific HMO utilizing microbes, mainly *Bifidobacterium* and *Bacteroides* species, interaction analysis between HMOs and such microbes is of particular interest. Such an interaction analysis recently revealed additional associations (Fig. 2) [20]. These findings lead to the hypothesis that only the presence of the right pairs of specific HMOs and bifidobacteria can support specific pathways affecting infant development.

Table 3. Associations reported for HMOs and brain development

Measure	Infant age (months)	Associated HMOs	
		Positive	Negative
ASQ score	(Preterm) 24	LNFP-III	
Cognitive development	24	2′-FL	
	6 and 18	2′-FL and 6′-SL	
Executive function	36	2′-FL and fucosyl-HMOs	Sialyl-HMOs
Language	12	3-FL, LNFP-II, and -V	
	<25	3′-SL	
	18	Fucosyl-HMOs	
		Sialyl-HMOs	
Social skills	12	LNT	
	12	6′-SL	
Gross motor	<12	3-FL	
Visually receptive	<12	3-FL	

Summarized based on findings from [20, 35–42].

Understanding Interaction Networks of Human Milk Oligosaccharides and Other Milk Components

Human milk is dynamic and diverse in composition, and HMOs are one such example of a dynamic and diverse compound family. As we have seen, maternal FUT2 and -3 genetic polymorphism determines part of the clusters seen among HMOs. Yet, correlation analysis also shows other HMO clusters (Fig. 1b). While cluster 5 mainly contains FUT3-dependent HMOs, the fucosylated HMOs in cluster 1 are both FUT2 and -3 dependent. Additionally, LNnT, a nonfucosylated HMO, also appears in cluster 1. Cluster 2 contains major sialylated LNT and LNT, which may be explained by the lower fucosylation of LNT, leading to higher sialylation. Interestingly, 3′-SL, which seems more universally present in almost all mammals, clusters with galactosyllactoses 3′-GL and 6′-GL. All three are also typically present in cow and other domestic animal milks (reviewed in [10]).

There is certainly more to learn from trying to understand HMO interaction networks and how these relate to clinical outcomes, directly or through the combination of specific gut microbiota, like infant-type *Bifidobacterium* species and *Bacteroides* species, which have the right biochemical pathways to utilize specific HMOs and to produce health-related biochemicals [20]. Figure 2 depicts associations identified by modeling interactions between individual HMOs and specific microbial taxa in relation to brain development-related outcome measures [20]. Shifting analysis more toward a systems biology approach, including the modeling of interaction networks not only among one compound group, like the HMOs, but also extending to other milk components, will allow us to expand our understanding of human milk biology and its benefits. As exemplified by Li et al. [45], joint analysis of multiple milk components underscores that many milk components work together to support infant development.

Conclusion

Human milk is a dynamic secretion of nutritive and bioactive components that support infant development during the first 6 months of age and beyond. The complexity of studying human milk is linked, in part, to the variation in its composition throughout lactation and in response to maternal factors, such as genetics and the environment, with HMO concentrations being a prime example. Evidence suggests that individual or structural groups of HMOs in human milk are associated with infant health, including somatic growth, immunity, and brain development. Emerging evidence indicates a role of the microbiome in mediating some effects of HMOs on infant health. A lack of consistency between observational studies in breastfed infants and limited effect sizes hampers our understanding of the true physiological relevance of the existing findings. Future advancements in the field of human milk biology require a more integrative approach to explore the interactions between human milk components and how such interactions drive the functionality and physiological benefits of human milk.

Acknowledgment

The authors kindly acknowledge Aristea Binia and Eline van der Beek for the careful review of this manuscript.

Conflict of Interest Statement

The authors are employees of Société des Produits Nestlé S.A., Switzerland.

Funding Sources

No funding was received.

Author Contributions

N.S. drafted the manuscript and C.R.M. completed, critically reviewed, and finalized the manuscript. Both authors reviewed and accept the final manuscript.

References

1 Dobzhansky T. Biology, molecular and organismic. JSTOR [Internet]. 1964 [cited 2023 Dec 15]; 4(4):443–52. https://doi.org/10.1093/icb/4.4.443.
2 Oftedal OT. The evolution of milk secretion and its ancient origins. Animal [Internet]. 2012 [cited 2023 Dec 7];6(3):355–68. https://doi.org/10.1017/S1751731111001935.
3 Christian P, Smith ER, Lee SE, Vargas AJ, Bremer AA, Raiten DJ. The need to study human milk as a biological system. Am J Clin Nutr. 2021;113(5): 1063–72. https://doi.org/10.1093/ajcn/nqab075.
4 World Health Organization. Global strategy for infant and young child feeding; 2003.
5 Victora CG, Bahl R, Barros AJD, França VA, Horton S, Krasevec J. Breastfeeding in the 21st century: epidemiology, mechanisms, and lifelong effects. Lancet [Internet]. 2016;387(10033): 2089–90. https://doi.org/10.1016/S0140-6736(16)30538-4.
6 Italianer MF, Naninck EFG, Roelants JA, van der Horst GTJ, Reiss IKM, van Goudoever JB, et al. Circadian variation in human milk composition, a systematic review. Nutrients. 2020;12(8):2328. https://doi.org/10.3390/nu12082328.
7 Karatas Z, Durmus Aydogdu S, Dinleyici EC, Colak O, Dogruel N. Breastmilk ghrelin, leptin, and fat levels changing foremilk to hindmilk: is that important for self-control of feeding? Eur J Pediatr. 2011;170(10):1273–80. https://doi.org/10.1007/s00431-011-1438-1.
8 Golan Y, Assaraf YG. Genetic and physiological factors affecting human milk production and composition. Nutrients. 2020;12(5):1500. https://doi.org/10.3390/nu12051500.

9 Fu Y, Liu X, Zhou B, Jiang AC, Chai L. An updated review of worldwide levels of docosahexaenoic and arachidonic acid in human breast milk by region. Public Health Nutr. 2016;19(15):2675–87. https://doi.org/10.1017/S1368980016000707.

10 Sprenger N, Tytgat HLP, Binia A, Austin S, Singhal A. Biology of human milk oligosaccharides: from basic science to clinical evidence. J Hum Nutr Diet. 2022; 35(2):280–99. https://doi.org/10.1111/jhn.12990.

11 Samuel TM, Binia A, de Castro CA, Thakkar SK, Billeaud C, Agosti M, et al. Impact of maternal characteristics on human milk oligosaccharide composition over the first 4 months of lactation in a cohort of healthy European mothers. Sci Rep. 2019;9(1):11767. https://doi.org/10.1038/s41598-019-48337-4.

12 Lefebvre G, Shevlyakova M, Charpagne A, Marquis J, Vogel M, Kirsten T, et al. Time of lactation and maternal fucosyltransferase genetic polymorphisms determine the variability in human milk oligosaccharides. Front Nutr. 2020;7:574459. https://doi.org/10.3389/fnut.2020.574459.

13 Austin S, De Castro CA, Sprenger N, Binia A, Affolter M, Garcia-Rodenas CL, et al. Human milk oligosaccharides in the milk of mothers delivering term versus preterm infants. Nutrients. 2019;11(6): 1282. https://doi.org/10.3390/nu11061282.

14 McGuire MK, Meehan CL, McGuire MA, Williams JE, Foster J, Sellen DW, et al. What's normal? Oligosaccharide concentrations and profiles in milk produced by healthy women vary geographically. Am J Clin Nutr. 2017;105(5):1086–100. https://doi.org/10.3945/ajcn.116.139980.

15 Davis JCC, Lewis ZT, Krishnan S, Bernstein RM, Moore SE, Prentice AM, et al. Growth and morbidity of Gambian infants are influenced by maternal milk oligosaccharides and infant gut microbiota. Sci Rep. 2017;7(1):40466. https://doi.org/10.1038/srep40466.

16 Biddulph C, Holmes M, Tran TD, Kuballa A, Davies PSW, Koorts P, et al. Associations between maternal nutrition and the concentrations of human milk oligosaccharides in a cohort of healthy Australian lactating women. Nutrients. 2023;15(9):2093. https://doi.org/10.3390/nu15092093.

17 Cochrane KM, Bone JN, Karakochuk CD, Bode L. Human milk oligosaccharide composition following supplementation with folic acid vs (6S)-5-methyltetrahydrofolic acid during pregnancy and mediation by human milk folate forms. Eur J Clin Nutr. 2024;78(4):351–5. https://doi.org/10.1038/s41430-023-01376-7.

18 Donald K, Finlay BB. Early-life interactions between the microbiota and immune system: impact on immune system development and atopic disease. Nat Rev Immunol. 2023;23(11):735–48. https://doi.org/10.1038/s41577-023-00874-w.

19 Dogra S, Chung C, Wang D, Sakwinska O, Colombo Mottaz S, Sprenger N. Nurturing the early life gut microbiome and immune maturation for long term health. Microorganisms. 2021;9(10):2110. https://doi.org/10.3390/microorganisms9102110.

20 Cho S, Samuel TM, Li T, Howell BR, Baluyot K, Hazlett HC, et al. Interactions between *Bifidobacterium* and *Bacteroides* and human milk oligosaccharides and their associations with infant cognition. Front Nutr. 2023;10:1216327. https://doi.org/10.3389/fnut.2023.1216327.

21 Olm MR, Dahan D, Carter MM, Merrill BD, Yu FB, Jain S, et al. Robust variation in infant gut microbiome assembly across a spectrum of lifestyles. Science. 2022;376(6598):1220–3. https://doi.org/10.1126/science.abj2972.

22 Loutet MG, Narimani A, Qamar H, Yonemitsu C, Pell LG, MA Al, et al. Associations between human milk oligosaccharides and infant growth in a Bangladeshi mother–infant cohort. Pediatr Res. 2023. https://doi.org/10.1038/s41390-023-02927-1.

23 Samuel TM, Hartweg M, Lebumfacil JD, B KatherineB, L RachelB, Estorninos EM, et al. Dynamics of human milk oligosaccharides in early lactation and relation with growth and appetitive traits of Filipino breastfed infants. Sci Rep. 2022; 12(1):17304. https://doi.org/10.1038/s41598-022-22244-7.

24 Charbonneau MR, O'Donnell D, Blanton LV, Totten SM, Davis JCC, Barratt MJ, et al. Sialylated milk oligosaccharides promote microbiota-dependent growth in models of infant undernutrition. Cell. 2016;164(5):859–71. https://doi.org/10.1016/j.cell.2016.01.024.

25 Cowardin CA, Ahern PP, Kung VL, Hibberd MC, Cheng J, Guruge JL, et al. Mechanisms by which sialylated milk oligosaccharides impact bone biology in a gnotobiotic mouse model of infant undernutrition. Proc Natl Acad Sci USA. 2019;116(24): 11988–96. https://doi.org/10.1073/pnas.1821770116.

26 Golden RK, Sutkus LT, Bauer LL, Donovan SM, Dilger RN. Determining the safety and efficacy of dietary supplementation with 3′-sialyllactose or 6′-sialyllactose on growth, tolerance, and brain sialic acid concentrations. Front Nutr. 2023;10:1278804. https://doi.org/10.3389/fnut.2023.1278804.

27 Binia A, Siegwald L, Sultana S, Shevlyakova M, Lefebvre G, Foata F, et al. The influence of *FUT2* and *FUT3* polymorphisms and nasopharyngeal microbiome on respiratory infections in breastfed Bangladeshi infants from the microbiota and health study. mSphere. 2021;6(6):e0068621. https://doi.org/10.1128/mSphere.00686-21.

28 Mottram L, Wiklund G, Larson G, Qadri F, Svennerholm AM. FUT2 non-secretor status is associated with altered susceptibility to symptomatic enterotoxigenic Escherichia coli infection in Bangladeshis. Sci Rep. 2017;7(1):10649. https://doi.org/10.1038/s41598-017-10854-5.

29 Zimmermann P, Messina N, Mohn WW, Finlay BB, Curtis N. Association between the intestinal microbiota and allergic sensitization, eczema, and asthma: a systematic review. J Allergy Clin Immunol. 2019;143(2): 467–85. https://doi.org/10.1016/j.jaci.2018.09.025.

30 Korpela K, Salonen A, Hickman B, Kunz C, Sprenger N, Kukkonen K, et al. Fucosylated oligosaccharides in mother's milk alleviate the effects of caesarean birth on infant gut microbiota. Sci Rep. 2018;8(1):13757. https://doi.org/10.1038/s41598-018-32037-6.

31 Sprenger N, Odenwald H, Kukkonen AK, Kuitunen M, Savilahti E, Kunz C. FUT2-dependent breast milk oligosaccharides and allergy at 2 and 5 years of age in infants with high hereditary allergy risk. Eur J Nutr. 2017;56(3):1293–301. https://doi.org/10.1007/s00394-016-1180-6.

32 Seppo AE, Autran CA, Bode L, Järvinen KM. Human milk oligosaccharides and development of cow's milk allergy in infants. J Allergy Clin Immunol. 2017;139(2):708–11.e5. https://doi.org/10.1016/j.jaci.2016.08.031.

33 Lodge CJ, Lowe AJ, Milanzi E, Bowatte G, Abramson MJ, Tsimiklis H, et al. Human milk oligosaccharide profiles and allergic disease up to 18 years. J Allergy Clin Immunol. 2021;147(3): 1041–8. https://doi.org/10.1016/j.jaci.2020.06.027.

34 Lian X, Zhang W, He-Yang J, Zhou X. Human milk oligosaccharide disialyllacto-n-tetraose protects human intestinal epithelium integrity and permeability against mast cell chymase-induced disruption by stabilizing ZO-1/FAK/P38 pathway of intestinal epithelial cell. Immunopharmacol Immunotoxicol. 2023;45(4):409–18. https://doi.org/10.1080/08923973.2022.2160730.

35 Rajhans P, Mainardi F, Austin S, Sprenger N, Deoni S, Hauser J, et al. The role of human milk oligosaccharides in myelination, socio-emotional and language development: observational data from breast-fed infants in the United States of America. Nutrients. 2023;15(21):4624. https://doi.org/10.3390/nu15214624.

36 Rozé JC, Hartweg M, Simon L, Billard H, Chen Y, Austin S, et al. Human milk oligosaccharides in breast milk and 2-year outcome in preterm infants: an exploratory analysis. Clin Nutr. 2022;41(9):1896–905. https://doi.org/10.1016/j.clnu.2022.07.024.

37 Berger PK, Plows JF, Jones RB, Alderete TL, Yonemitsu C, Poulsen M, et al. Human milk oligosaccharide 2'-fucosyllactose links feedings at 1 month to cognitive development at 24 months in infants of normal and overweight mothers. PLoS One. 2020;15(2):e0228323. https://doi.org/10.1371/journal.pone.0228323.

38 Willemsen Y, Beijers R, Gu F, Vasquez AA, Schols HA, de Weerth C. Fucosylated human milk oligosaccharides during the first 12 postnatal weeks are associated with better executive functions in toddlers. Nutrients. 2023;15(6):1463. https://doi.org/10.3390/nu15061463.

39 Ferreira ALL, Alves-Santos NH, Freitas-Costa NC, Santos PPT, Batalha MA, Figueiredo ACC, et al. Associations between human milk oligosaccharides at 1 Month and infant development throughout the first year of life in a Brazilian cohort. J Nutr. 2021;151(11):3543–54. https://doi.org/10.1093/jn/nxab271.

40 Jorgensen JM, Young R, Ashorn P, Ashorn U, Chaima D, Davis JC, et al. Associations of human milk oligosaccharides and bioactive proteins with infant growth and development among Malawian mother-infant dyads. Am J Clin Nutr. 2021;113(1):209–20. https://doi.org/10.1093/ajcn/nqaa272.

41 Cho S, Zhu Z, Li T, Baluyot K, Howell BR, Hazlett HC, et al. Human milk 3'-Sialyllactose is positively associated with language development during infancy. Am J Clin Nutr. 2021; 114(2):588–97. https://doi.org/10.1093/ajcn/nqab103.

42 Oliveros E, Martín MJ, Torres-Espínola FJ, Segura-Moreno MT, Ramírez M, Santos A, et al. Human milk levels of 2´-fucosyllactose and 6´-sialyllactose are positively associated with infant neurodevelopment and are not impacted by maternal BMI or diabetic status. J Nutr Food Sci. 2021; 4(1):024.

43 Hauser J, Pisa E, Arias Vásquez A, Tomasi F, Traversa A, Chiodi V, et al. Sialylated human milk oligosaccharides program cognitive development through a non-genomic transmission mode. Mol Psychiatry. 2021;26(7):2854–71. https://doi.org/10.1038/s41380-021-01054-9.

44 Sprenger N, Duncan PI. Sialic acid utilization. Adv Nutr. 2012;3(3):392S–397S. https://doi.org/10.3945/an.111.001479.

45 Li T, Samuel TM, Zhu Z, Howell B, Cho S, Baluyot K, et al. Joint analyses of human milk fatty acids, phospholipids, and choline in association with cognition and temperament traits during the first 6 months of life. Front Nutr. 2022;9. https://doi.org/10.3389/fnut.2022.919769.

Norbert Sprenger
Gastrointestinal Health Department
Nestlé Institute of Health Sciences
Route du Jorat 57, Vers-chez-les-Blanc
1000 Lausanne 26, Switzerland
Norbert.Sprenger@rdls.nestle.com

Published online: November 15, 2024

Szajewska H, Neu J, Shamir R, Wong G, Prentice AM (eds): Shaping the Future with Nutrition. Nestle Nutr Inst Workshop Ser. Basel, Karger, 2024, vol 100, pp 71–80 (DOI: 10.1159/000540137)

Nutrition for the Sick Preterm: Can We Make It More Precise?

Josef Neu

Department of Pediatrics, Division of Neonatology, University of Florida, Gainesville, FL, USA

Abstract

In the early era of neonatal intensive care (about 5–6 decades ago), most nutritional approaches were based largely on the physician's intuition, previous experience, and patient's signs and symptoms. This resulted in a large heterogeneity of diagnostic, preventative, and therapeutic measures. More recently, evidence-based approaches, such as data reviews and clinical trials, form the foundation for nutritional guidelines used in most Neonatal Intensive Care Unit (NICUs). These are derived from population statistics aimed toward the average and, thereby, meet the needs of many of these infants, but because of the extreme heterogeneity of the preterm population, they marginalize others. Helpful scoring programs are now available to identify malnutrition in populations of preterm infants using defined indicators. However, similar to growth curves, they do not provide proactive guidance. Newly developed precision-based approaches using algorithms and predictive analytics based on artificial intelligence (AI) and machine learning (ML) will provide for a priori-based preventative approaches. It is likely that these will employ technologies that cluster infants into different risk categories that can then be investigated mechanistically with multiomic integrations that provide mechanistic interactions and provide clues to biomarkers that can be used for the discovery of biomarkers that can be utilized for the development of preventative strategies.

Introduction and Historical Perspective

The history of neonatal intensive care is fraught with struggles as to how to best nourish preterm infants for the best possible outcomes. Figure 1 depicts the eras of medicine: where we have been, where we are now, and the likely future of nutrition in NICU care.

During the early era of modern neonatal intensive care, the 1970s, up to the last decade, it was common practice to withhold parenteral and enteral nutrition in preterm infants for the fear of causing metabolic imbalances and inducing intestinal injury. These infants have very low energy and protein stores and are, thus, highly susceptible to undernutrition and catabolism. In the early era of neonatal intensive care (about 5–6 decades ago), many nutritional approaches were largely based on the physician's intuition, previous experience, and patient's signs and symptoms. Not all physicians had similar previous experiences and there were numerous different approaches to care. This resulted in heterogeneity of diagnostic, preventative, and therapeutic measures.

More recently, evidence-based approaches, such as retrospective data reviews, cohort studies, and prospective randomized clinical trials, have begun to form the foundation for nutritional guidelines used in most NICUs. These are derived from population statistics and lead to recommendations aimed toward the average of the population and, thereby, meet the needs of many of these infants, but because of the extreme heterogeneity of the preterm population, they marginalize others. In addition, helpful scoring programs have been developed to identify malnutrition in populations of preterm infants using defined indicators [1, 2], but, like growth curves, they do very little to provide proactive guidance.

There is currently a trend toward precision-based approaches using algorithms and predictive analytics based on artificial intelligence (AI) and machine learning (ML) that provide for a priori-based preventative approaches, which will be reviewed.

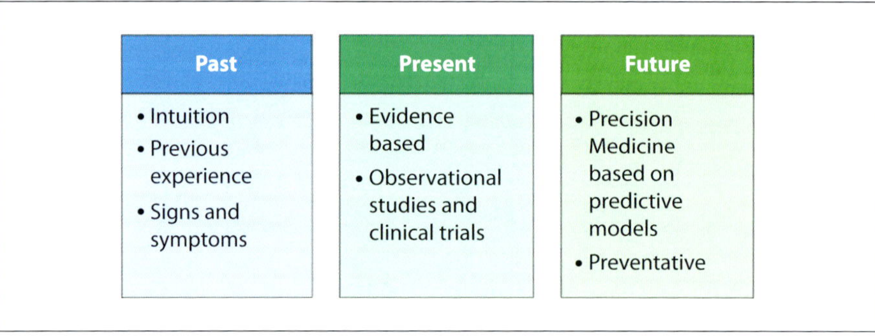

Fig. 1. Eras of medicine.

Problems with Current Approaches

What are the problems with our previous and current approaches to nutrition for preterm infants? One major consideration is that even short periods of undernutrition in these highly vulnerable infants can result in catabolism during a time when the infant should be undergoing rapid growth and brain development. The gestational age for many of the infants cared for in modern neonatology is considerably lower than that in previous decades, and a 23-week gestational age preterm infant has different nutritional requirements than the one born at 32 weeks of gestation.

Withholding parenteral and enteral nutrition for prolonged periods with subsequent extremely slow advancement ("starvation") [3] in neonatal intensive care has fortunately become less common. Evidence-based approaches have led to guideline-based strategies for nutritional optimization [4, 5]. However, neonatal intensive care has been evolving and guidelines based on population statistics rather than individual needs will result in faulty nutritional delivery to many of these infants for several reasons:

1. Current neonatal intensive care is experiencing survival of preterm infants to 22 weeks of gestational age [6]. Attempting to meet the nutritional needs of these extremely immature infants using the same guidelines as for those born at 34 weeks presents a conundrum since the needs across this spectrum differ markedly [7]. The 22-week preterm has nearly no energy stores available in the form of fat and, thus, cutting off nutrition from the mother's placenta puts the infant at high risk for both short- and long-term adverse outcomes if not immediately nourished after birth [3].
2. Population-based studies suggest that many preterm infants can have their enteral feedings safely advanced at rates of up to 30 mL/kg per day [8–10]. When enteral feeding is advanced at rates up to 30 mL/kg per day, many preterm infants will rapidly attain adequate fluid volume and basic nutrients, obviating the need for prolonged parenteral nutrition with its associated adverse consequences [11]. Despite these improvements, many preterm infants clearly cannot tolerate this rate of advancement. Feedings are withheld, especially in those with the lowest gestational age, for unsubstantiated reasons, such as gastric residuals, use of medications, such as indomethacin and blood transfusions. Our group has helped debunk some of these practices (gastric residuals) [12–14], and withholding feedings during blood transfusions [15], and has been involved with numerous studies related to the feeding composition and strategies in the neonate [4, 16–22]. Which subsets of preterm infants may be advanced at a more rapid rate and what composition of feedings they will most likely tolerate is a major gap in our nutritional strategies.

3. Intravenous feedings also present a conundrum. Aiming toward amino acid infusions of 3–4 g/kg per day [23] and lipid infusions of 3 g/kg per day [24], the levels derived by the fetus in utero, seems to be the correct approach for many of these infants, but may result in metabolic imbalances and sepsis in certain susceptible infants [25–27]. This is especially problematic in infants receiving antenatal steroids [28] and/or who were born intrauterine growth restricted (IUGR) [29]. Major differences are seen in the metabolomic profiles of cord blood in infants who are IUGR compared to those who are appropriate for gestational age (AGA) [29]. These infants likely have different nutritional requirements and metabolic responses to certain nutritional regimens than AGA infants.
4. In addition to undernutrition, overcompensating for faltering on growth curves to promote "catch-up growth" is also concerning. Some preterm infants who have undergone intrauterine growth restriction (IUGR) have suffered in-utero malnutrition and applying the same approach used for appropriate for gestational age (AGA) infants is associated with long-term adverse consequences, such as obesity, diabetes, and hypertension, the so-called "metabolic syndrome" [30–33].
5. Refeeding syndrome following preterm birth, especially in IUGR infants, necessitates a different nutritional approach, but this is not yet defined [34].
6. Early nutritional practices also affect the microbiome differentially, even among identical twins [35]. This can affect immune development, as well as the metabolome and the closely related epigenome, aberrations to which may not only have lifelong, but also transgenerational consequences [36].
7. Sexual, racial, and socioeconomic factors also play roles that beg for personalization.

Thus, in the early era of neonatal intensive care, there was considerable heterogeneity of care. Many infants were not provided with intravenous lipids for days after their birth because they had hyperbilirubinemia and there was concern that providing lipids would lead to the displacement of bilirubin from albumin, leading to kernicterus. Preterm infants were not enterally fed for days and sometimes weeks because there was concern that their intestinal tracts could not tolerate feedings, and this would dispose to intestinal necrosis. In the more recent era, evidence-based approaches that included studies of populations of infants have provided evidence of what nutritional approaches provide benefits or harm to the average part of the population, and this has led to nutritional guidelines for enteral feedings, composition of parenteral nutrition, and what the actual nutritional needs of most of these infants are. These evidence-based techniques have provided guidance using tools, such as growth curves, which have been a breakthrough in how we nourish infants. However, as seen in Figure 2, growth curves also have shortfalls.

- If we see growth faltering, is it already too late?
- Do we need indicators that help prevent this or should we stick to the old Gaussian statistics aiming for the mean?
- Can we predict this before it occurs?
- More precise nutrition should be possible.

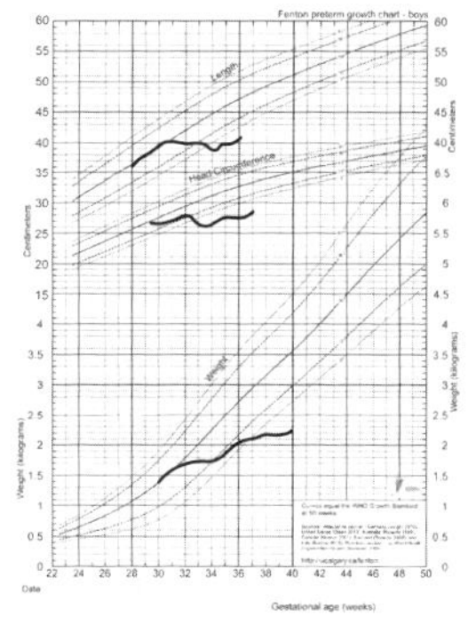

Fig. 2. Current monitoring of nutrition. Source: Fenton TR, Kim JH. A systematic review and meta-analysis to revise the Fenton growth chart for preterm infants. BMC Pediatr. 2013;13:59. https://doi.org/10.1186/1471-2431-13-59 [47].

Once growth faltering or malnutrition is noticed using growth curves, this will raise concern, but it may already be too late for meaningful interventions for many of these infants who are highly sensitive to nutritional deficiencies.

Problems with Current Guideline-Based Approaches

As previously mentioned, guideline-based nutritional approaches that rely on evidence-based studies have provided major advances over previous intuition-based approaches for nourishing these infants. However, preterm infants are highly heterogeneous, and the suitability of guideline-based approaches is being questioned [37, 38]. One guideline does not fit all preterm nutritional needs. For example, an extremely preterm infant born at 22 weeks' gestational age has requirements that differ markedly from one born at 32 weeks' gestation [7]; an infant born to a mother with severe obesity differs metabolically and has different nutritional needs compared to an infant born to a lean mother [39]; an infant receiving antibiotics either prenatally, perinatally, or immediately postnatally is likely to have a microbiome, metabolome, and proteome that differs from an infant not exposed to antibiotics and, thus, will respond to nutrients differently than one not exposed to antibiotics [40]. Neonates with severe in-utero growth restriction are clearly different metabolically with early patterns of glucose intolerance, insulin resistance, catabolite accumulation, disrupted amino acid metabolism, and abnormal fetal liver function [41]. Recent data suggest that sex also plays a role in the nutritional needs of preterm infants [42]. Numerous other factors can alter a preterm infant's nutritional needs [43].

Nutritional guidelines using a "one-size-fits-all" approach may malnourish many infants and dispose them toward adverse outcomes, such as necrotizing enterocolitis (NEC), retinopathy of prematurity (ROP), bronchopulmonary dysplasia (BPD), late-onset sepsis (LOS), and growth failure (GF) (Fig. 3). Overnutrition or "catch-up growth" can lead to adverse lifelong and even transgenerational consequences, which include the metabolic syndrome [44].

This begs for a different nutritional approach in these infants compared to those born appropriate for gestational age. A proactive, precision-based approach directed toward the personal needs of preterm infants that transcends a one-size-fits-all guideline-based approach is urgently needed. Figure 4 illustrates the potential approach for future studies.

A promising approach includes machine learning (ML) and multiomics. Machine learning provides the opportunity for the high-resolution classification of infants at the greatest risk and for predictive analytics for preemptive precision-based approaches initiated very early after birth. Multiomic integrations provide mechanistic characterization and provide the opportunity for the discovery of biomarkers that can be applied for precisely guiding nutritional interventions in individual infants.

Our recently published study indicates their feasibility and is an initial step toward such an approach [45]. This study utilized clinical and microbiome datasets from four different sources in the US and UK. Machine learning methods utilized clinical indicators for growth failure prediction; then, these were extended to include longitudinal microbiome analysis. This study demonstrated that a hierarchical classifier using a subset of the microbial taxa combined with clinical features has the potential to be utilized for growth

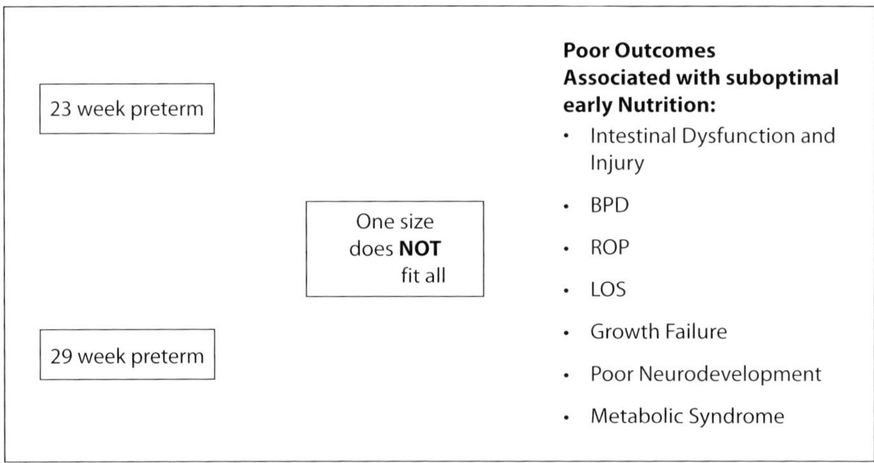

Fig. 3. Why personalized nutrition?

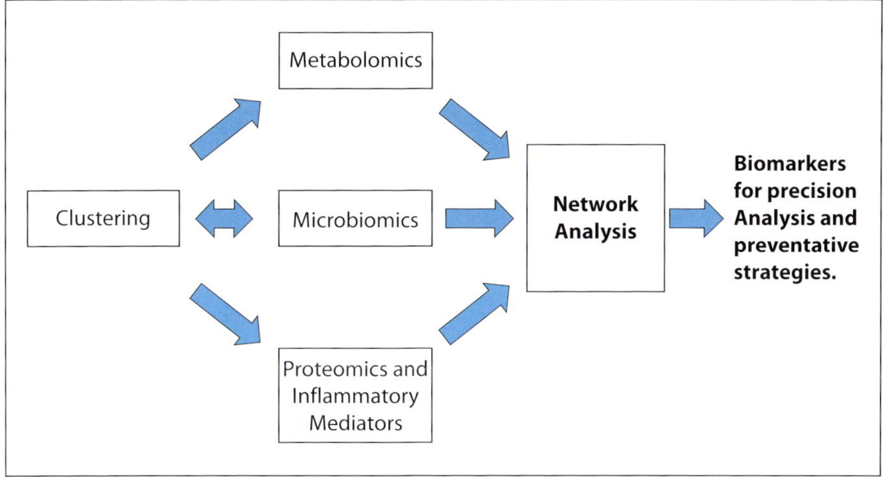

Fig. 4. Proposed pathway for the future.

failure prediction. However, considerable refinement is needed, which is the goal of this research.

Research will classify preterm infants into clusters with different clinical severity scores and discover causal mechanisms for nutritional inadequacies within these clusters using integrated multiomics. Specific predictive biomarkers will be established from these mechanistic studies that will enable early nutritional interventions specifically tailored for individual preterm infants. We anticipate results that lead to methods for the prevention of devastating outcomes in preterm infants while the infant is hospitalized, enhance lifelong health, and influence outcomes for future generations [36, 46].

Conclusion

The rapidly emerging fields of artificial intelligence and multiomics are highly applicable to various problems we see in perinatology and neonatal intensive care. Predictive analytics using supervised and unsupervised machine learning techniques, as well as closely related neural network technologies, will help in the categorization of infants with specialized needs and who may be on a path toward either early or late-onset pathologies. With such recognition, we should be able to intervene early to prevent these problems from occurring.

Similarly, we are beginning to make significant strides in precision nutrition. Previous studies show interesting associations between giving or withholding certain nutrients and clinical outcomes. However, the mechanisms and causal nature of these associations are not well understood. These are amenable to analysis by newly developing technologies, such as multiomics and artificial intelligence. These will be applied in the future to better understand mechanisms and to provide personalized nutrition for both mothers and their infants.

The future in these areas is very exciting but we will need to closely collaborate in highly functioning teams that include clinicians, basic scientists, engineers, bioinformaticians, mathematicians, and other highly skilled individuals.

Conflict of Interest Statement

The author is a member of the Global Nestlé Nutrition Institute Scientific Council, serves on the Scientific Advisory Boards for Arla, Medela, and Astarte, has a research grant from Infant Bacterial Therapeutics, and is a consultant for Siolta Therapeutics.

Funding Sources

The author received lecture honoraria and travel reimbursement from Nestlé Nutrition Institute.

Author Contributions

Josef Neu is the sole author.

References

1 Goldberg DL, Becker PJ, Brigham K, Carlson S, Fleck L, Gollins L, et al. Identifying malnutrition in preterm and neonatal populations: recommended indicators. J Acad Nutr Diet. 2018;118(9):1571–82. https://doi.org/10.1016/j.jand.2017.10.006.

2 Izquierdo RM, Aldecoa-Bilbao V, Balcells Esponera C, Del Rey Hurtado de Mendoza B, Iriondo Sanz M, Iglesias-Platas I. Applying methods for postnatal growth assessment in the clinical setting: evaluation in a longitudinal cohort of very preterm infants. Nutrients. 2019;11(11):2772. https://doi.org/10.3390/nu11112772.

3 Neu J. Is it time to stop starving premature infants? J Perinatol. 2009;29(6):399–400. https://doi.org/10.1038/jp.2009.46.

4 Raiten DJ, Steiber AL, Carlson SE, Griffin I, Anderson D, Hay WW, Jr., et al. Working group reports: evaluation of the evidence to support practice guidelines for nutritional care of preterm infants-the Pre-B Project. Am J Clin Nutr. 2016; 103(2):648S–78S. https://doi.org/10.3945/ajcn.115.117309.

5 Torrazza RM, Neu J. Evidence-based guidelines for optimization of nutrition for the very low birthweight infant. NeoReviews. 2013;14(7): e340–49. https://doi.org/10.1542/neo.14-7-e340.

6 Yanagisawa T, Nakamura T, Kokubo M. Prognosis of 22- and 23-gestational-week-old infants at our facility: a retrospective cohort study. Am J Perinatol. 2024;41(5):660–68. https://doi.org/10.1055/a-1779-4032.

7 Patton L, de la Cruz D, Neu J. Gastrointestinal and feeding issues for infants <25 weeks of gestation. Semin Perinatol. 2022;46(1):151546. https://doi.org/10.1016/j.semperi.2021.151546.

8 Dorling J, Abbott J, Berrington J, Bosiak B, Bowler U, Boyle E, et al. Controlled trial of two incremental milk-feeding rates in preterm infants. N Engl J Med. 2019;381(15):1434–43. https://doi.org/10.1056/NEJMoa1816654.

9 Alshaikh B, Dharel D, Yusuf K, Singhal N. Early total enteral feeding in stable preterm infants: a systematic review and meta-analysis. J Matern Fetal Neonatal Med. 2021;34(9):1479–86. http://doi.org/10.1080/14767058.2019.1637848.
10 Rayyis SF, Ambalavanan N, Wright L, Carlo WA. Randomized trial of "slow" versus "fast" feed advancements on the incidence of necrotizing enterocolitis in very low birth weight infants. J Pediatr. 1999;134(3):293–7. https://doi.org/10.1016/s0022-3476(99)70452-x.
11 National Guideline A. Predictors of enteral feeding success: neonatal parenteral nutrition: evidence review A1. London: National Institute for Health and Care Excellence (UK); 2020.
12 Parker LA, Weaver M, Murgas Torrazza RJ, Shuster J, Li N, Krueger C, et al. Effect of gastric residual evaluation on enteral intake in extremely preterm infants: a randomized clinical trial. JAMA Pediatr. 2019;173(6):534–43. https://doi.org/10.1001/jamapediatrics.2019.0800.
13 Parker LA, Weaver M, Murgas Torrazza RJ, Shuster J, Li N, Krueger C, et al. Effect of aspiration and evaluation of gastric residuals on intestinal inflammation, bleeding, and gastrointestinal peptide level. J Pediatr. 2020;217:165–71.e2. https://doi.org/10.1016/j.jpeds.2019.10.036.
14 Torrazza RM, Parker LA, Li Y, Talaga E, Shuster J, Neu J. The value of routine evaluation of gastric residuals in very low birth weight infants. J Perinatol. 2015;35(1):57–60. https://doi.org/10.1038/jp.2014.147.
15 Sharma R, Kraemer DF, Torrazza RM, Mai V, Neu J, Shuster JJ, et al. Packed red blood cell transfusion is not associated with increased risk of necrotizing enterocolitis in premature infants. J Perinatol. 2014;34(11):858–62. https://doi.org/10.1038/jp.2014.59.
16 Chang LL, Wynn JL, Pacella MJ, Rossignol CC, Banadera F, Alviedo N, et al. Enteral feeding as an adjunct to hypothermia in neonates with hypoxic-ischemic encephalopathy. Neonatology. 2018;113(4):347–52. https://doi.org/10.1159/000487848.
17 Cortez J, Makker K, Kraemer DF, Neu J, Sharma R, Hudak ML. Maternal milk feedings reduce sepsis, necrotizing enterocolitis and improve outcomes of premature infants. J Perinatol. 2018;38(1):71–4. https://doi.org/10.1038/jp.2017.149.
18 Roze JC, Ancel PY, Lepage P, Martin-Marchand L, Al Nabhani Z, Delannoy J, et al. Nutritional strategies and gut microbiota composition as risk factors for necrotizing enterocolitis in very-preterm infants. Am J Clin Nutr. 2017;106(3):821–30. https://doi.org/10.3945/ajcn.117.152967.
19 Cacho NT, Parker LA, Neu J. Necrotizing enterocolitis and human milk feeding: a systematic review. Clin Perinatol. 2017;44(1):49–67. https://doi.org/10.1016/j.clp.2016.11.009.
20 Neu J, Bradley CL, Ding ZY, Tucker HN, Berseth CL. Feeding the preterm infant: opportunities and challenges of bringing science to the bedside. J Pediatr. 2013;162(3 Suppl l):S101–6. https://doi.org/10.1016/j.jpeds.2012.11.059.
21 Wiedmeier JE, Joss-Moore LA, Lane RH, Neu J. Early postnatal nutrition and programming of the preterm neonate. Nutr Rev. 2011;69(2):76–82. https://doi.org/10.1111/j.1753-4887.2010.00370.x.
22 Neu J. Gastrointestinal maturation and implications for infant feeding. Early Hum Dev. 2007;83(12):767–75. https://doi.org/10.1016/j.earlhumdev.2007.09.009.
23 Denne SC, Poindexter BB. Evidence supporting early nutritional support with parenteral amino acid infusion. Semin Perinatol. 2007;31(2):56–60. https://doi.org/10.1053/j.semperi.2007.02.005.
24 Salama GS, Kaabneh MA, Almasaeed MN, Alquran M. Intravenous lipids for preterm infants: a review. Clin Med Insights Pediatr. 2015;9:25–36. https://doi.org/10.4137/CMPed.S21161.
25 Guellec I, Gascoin G, Beuchee A, Boubred F, Tourneux P, Ramful D, et al. Biological impact of recent guidelines on parenteral nutrition in preterm infants. J Pediatr Gastroenterol Nutr. 2015;61(6):605–9. https://doi.org/10.1097/MPG.0000000000000898.
26 Clark RH, Chace DH, Spitzer AR, Pediatrix Amino Acid Study Group. Effects of two different doses of amino acid supplementation on growth and blood amino acid levels in premature neonates admitted to the neonatal intensive care unit: a randomized, controlled trial. Pediatrics. 2007;120(6):1286–96. https://doi.org/10.1542/peds.2007-0545.
27 Moltu SJ, Strømmen K, Blakstad EW, Almaas AN, Westerberg AC, Brække K, et al. Enhanced feeding in very-low-birth-weight infants may cause electrolyte disturbances and septicemia – a randomized, controlled trial. Clin Nutr. 2013;32(2):207–12. https://doi.org/10.1016/j.clnu.2012.09.004.
28 de Pipaón MS, VanBeek RH, Zimmermann LJ, Wattimena DJ, Quero J, Sauer PJ. Effects of antenatal steroids on protein metabolism in preterm infants on the first day of life. J Pediatr. 2004;144(1):75–80. https://doi.org/10.1016/j.jpeds.2003.10.017.
29 Moros G, Boutsikou T, Fotakis C, Iliodromiti Z, Sokou R, Katsila T, et al. Insights into intrauterine growth restriction based on maternal and umbilical cord blood metabolomics. Sci Rep. 2021;11(1):7824. https://doi.org/10.1038/s41598-021-87323-7.
30 Toftlund LH, Halken S, Agertoft L, Zachariassen G. Early nutrition and signs of metabolic syndrome at

6 y of age in children born very preterm. Am J Clin Nutr. 2018;107(5):717–24. https://doi.org/10.1093/ajcn/nqy015.
31 Lapillonne A, Griffin IJ. Feeding preterm infants today for later metabolic and cardiovascular outcomes. J Pediatr. 2013;162(3 Suppl l):S7–16. https://doi.org/10.1016/j.jpeds.2012.11.048.
32 Markopoulou P, Papanikolaou E, Analytis A, Zoumakis E, Siahanidou T. Preterm birth as a risk factor for metabolic syndrome and cardiovascular disease in adult life: a systematic review and meta-analysis. J Pediatr. 2019;210:69–80.e5. https://doi.org/10.1016/j.jpeds.2019.02.041.
33 Parkinson JRC, Hyde MJ, Gale C, Santhakumaran S, Modi N. Preterm birth and the metabolic syndrome in adult life: a systematic review and meta-analysis. Pediatrics. 2013;131(4):e1240–63. https://doi.org/10.1542/peds.2012-2177.
34 Cormack BE, Jiang Y, Harding JE, Crowther CA, Bloomfield FH, ProVIDe Trial Group. Neonatal refeeding syndrome and clinical outcome in extremely low-birth-weight babies: secondary cohort analysis from the ProVIDe trial. JPEN J Parenter Enteral Nutr. 2021;45(1):65–78. https://doi.org/10.1002/jpen.1934.
35 Berry SE, Valdes AM, Drew DA, Asnicar F, Mazidi M, Wolf J, et al. Human postprandial responses to food and potential for precision nutrition. Nat Med. 2020;26(6):964–73. https://doi.org/10.1038/s41591-020-0934-0.
36 Indrio F, Martini S, Francavilla R, Corvaglia L, Cristofori F, Mastrolia SA, et al. Epigenetic matters: the link between early nutrition, microbiome, and long-term health development. Front Pediatr. 2017;5: 178. https://doi.org/10.3389/fped.2017.00178.
37 Young A, Beattie RM, Johnson MJ. Optimising growth in very preterm infants: reviewing the evidence. Arch Dis Child Fetal Neonatal Ed. 2023; 108(1):2–9. https://doi.org/10.1136/archdischild-2021-322892.
38 Webbe J, Uthaya S, Modi N. Nutrition for the micro preemie: beyond milk. Semin Fetal Neonatal Med 2022;27(3):101344. https://doi.org/10.1016/j.siny.2022.101344.
39 Robinson DT, Josefson J, Van Horn L. Considerations for preterm human milk feedings when caring for mothers who are overweight or obese. Adv Neonatal Care. 2019;19(5):361–70. https://doi.org/10.1097/ANC.0000000000000650.
40 Luo P, Zhang K, Chen Y, Geng X, Wu T, Li L, et al. Antenatal antibiotic exposure affects enteral feeding, body growth, and neonatal infection in preterm infants: a retrospective study. Front Pediatr. 2021;9:750058. https://doi.org/10.3389/fped.2021.750058.
41 Priante E, Verlato G, Giordano G, Stocchero M, Visentin S, Mardegan V, et al. Intrauterine growth restriction: new insight from the metabolomic approach. Metabolites. 2019;9(11):267. https://doi.org/10.3390/metabo9110267.
42 Tottman AC, Bloomfield FH, Cormack BE, Harding JE, Taylor J, Alsweiler JM. Sex-specific relationships between early nutrition and neurodevelopment in preterm infants. Pediatr Res. 2020; 87(5):872–8. https://doi.org/10.1038/s41390-019-0695-y.
43 Raiten DJ, Steiber AL, Hand RK. Executive summary: evaluation of the evidence to support practice guidelines for nutritional care of preterm infants-the Pre-B Project. Am J Clin Nutr. 2016; 103(2):599s–605s. https://doi.org/10.3945/ajcn.115.124222.
44 Gounaris A, Sokou R, Panagiotounakou P, Grivea IN. It is time for a universal nutrition policy in very preterm neonates during the neonatal period? Comment on: "Applying methods for postnatal growth assessment in the clinical setting: evaluation in a longitudinal cohort of very preterm infants" Nutrients 2019, 11, 2772. Nutrients. 2020;12(4): 980. https://doi.org/10.3390/nu12040980.
45 Lugo-Martinez J, Xu S, Levesque J, Gallagher D, Parker LA, Neu J, et al. Integrating longitudinal clinical and microbiome data to predict growth faltering in preterm infants. J Biomed Inform. 2022;128:104031
46 Patel MS, Srinivasan M. Metabolic programming in the immediate postnatal life. Ann Nutr Metab. 2011;58(Suppl 2):18–28. https://doi.org/10.1159/000328040.
47 Fenton TR, Kim JH. A systematic review and meta-analysis to revise the Fenton growth chart for preterm infants. BMC Pediatr. 2013;13:59. https://doi.org/10.1186/1471-2431-13-59.

Josef Neu
Department of Pediatrics/Division of Neonatology
University of Florida
1600 SW Archer Road
Gainesville, FL 32610, USA
neuj@peds.ulf.edu

Published online: November 15, 2024

Szajewska H, Neu J, Shamir R, Wong G, Prentice AM (eds): Shaping the Future with Nutrition. Nestle Nutr Inst Workshop Ser. Basel, Karger, 2024, vol 100, pp 81–89 (DOI: 10.1159/000540134)

Better Early: Critical Windows in Brain and Cognitive Development

Bernadette C. Benitez

Section of Developmental and Behavioral Pediatrics, Department of Pediatrics, Makati Medical Center, Makati, Philippines

Abstract

The first 3 years of life are when dynamic neurodevelopmental processes unfold. This is marked by sensitive or critical windows of opportunities, during which the young brain is both adaptable and vulnerable. Factors like nutrient deficiencies and inadequate environmental stimulation are more likely to negatively impact early brain development, especially when necessary and timely identification and intervention are not put in place. The benefits of adequate nutrition, especially breastfeeding during the first 1,000 days, cannot be overemphasized. Evidences from newer modalities of research, utilizing magnetic resonance imaging, continue to point to the significant influence of early life nutrition on early brain development, particularly myelination. Paradigms show that a child's physical growth, activity, and overall health influence the way he interacts with the environment, laying the scaffolds for brain development and learning. Current evidences show how the recent pandemic has impacted this very foundation, affecting children's nutrition, behavior, and development. There is a renewed call for pediatricians and other healthcare practitioners in clinics and communities to more ardently screen, monitor for, and provide proper advice for concerns regarding growth and development during the first 3 years of life to help mitigate the impact of current global events on children's potential to adapt, learn, and be productive adults in the future.

Introduction

Vital to every child's development is how their brain grows and matures in the early years of life, beginning in conception to about the third year, which is the most sensitive period to both positive protective factors and toxic stressors.

Critical Windows in Brain and Cognitive Development

Current scientific and clinical evidence shows how the intricate ecosystem of nature and nurture variables interacts and shapes early brain development. Factors like one's genetic blueprint and environmental experiences support the basic foundations of the brain's architecture, which is core to a child's learning ability, their overall physical and mental health, their ability to adapt and be resilient, and their capacity to become a self-sustaining adult capable of contributing positively to their family and community [1].

The first 3 years of life is the period when dynamic neurodevelopmental processes take place and neuroplasticity is at its peak. The complex process begins with neurogenesis or the creation of single brain-cell units or neurons which then migrate to their predisposed locations along with their appendages, allowing these to link with other neurons in the process of synaptogenesis. Myelination takes place to facilitate effective and efficient communication among neurons, allowing the creation of more than a million connections every second. These complex processes facilitate the acquisition of sensory perception and processing skills that proceeds to language and cognitive development and then further moves on to the learning of higher-order thinking skills and executive function [2, 3]. These neurodevelopmental processes are sensitive to nutrition and environmental factors that are stimulating and nurturing. If children fail to get what they need during the most critical years of early childhood, the impact on their lives and futures is enormous [4].

Learning is intimately related to how neurodevelopmental processes proceed, more specifically with myelination, which is considered a cornerstone of cognitive development. Advances in neuroimaging have allowed workers in this field to have a closer look at how myelin development impacts early milestones and subsequent learning among young children. Using magnetic resonance imaging, Pujol et al. [5] demonstrated the relationship of myelin development from 0 to 3 years of age with how children acquire speech and language. They demonstrated that once a rapid myelination phase is attained in the language centers of the brain, enhancement of vocabulary and language performance followed suit.

Recent researches utilizing more advanced neuroimaging techniques developed in the past decade have gathered interesting data on developmental myelination and the influence of early life nutrition on myelin volume and subsequent cognitive scores in early childhood.

In a study by Deoni et al. [6], the researchers investigated early nutritional influences on longitudinal infant- and child-brain development in a naturalistic setting. Using MRI images of healthy, typically developing 3-month- to 9-year-old children, they found that exclusive breastfeeding for at least 3 months was not only associated with improved myelination throughout the brain by the age of 2, but also that breastfed children demonstrated improved cognitive abilities compared to children fed infant alone. Statistically significant differences across both verbal and nonverbal quotients were noted for both groups, and these changes, observed as early as 18 months, persisted until early childhood [6].

Taking these findings further, a two-center, randomized controlled trial looked at the efficacy of an experimental formula on longitudinal myelination and cognitive and behavioral development from birth to 2 years of age. The experimental formula (EF) was a blend of DHA, AA, iron, vitamin B12, folic acid, and sphingomyelin from a uniquely processed whey protein concentrate enriched with alpha-lactalbumin and phospholipids, while the control formula (CF) had a similar nutrient matrix but at lower, regulatory-compliant levels with the standard whey protein concentrate. A nonrandomized reference group of breastfed infants were also included. The study spanned a 12-month intervention period. Using MRI during natural nonsedated sleep, the researchers compared the EF versus CF group across six visits (at 3, 6, 9, 12, 18, and 24 months) using the following outcomes: myelination, measured by the myelin water fraction, and cognitive abilities, as measured by Bayley III, socio-emotional development, sleep, and safety.

Preliminary outcomes from a staged statistical analysis at 6 months showed observed significant differences in myelin structure, volume, and rate of myelination in favor of the investigational myelin blend at 3 and 6 months of life. The effects were demonstrated for whole-brain myelin and for the cerebellar, parietal, occipital, and temporal regions, known to be functionally involved in sensory, motor, and language skills [7]. Unpublished data at the end of the 24-month study period showed that the EF nutrient blend increased myelin up to 24 months of life where the whole-brain myelin water fraction was seen to be significantly higher in the experimental group than that in the control. There were also enhanced differences in the white matter in the frontal, temporal, and parietal areas which may play vital roles in the development of motor, executive function, and language skills. Along with this, the gray matter volume was also observed to have significantly increased. Other observed outcomes include fewer night awakenings at 6 months, longer daytime sleep and motor skills acquisition at 12 months, and reduced social fearfulness at 24 months.

These findings are among many of the recent scientific evidences that demonstrate the positive influence of adequate early nutrition on brain development. However, as previously stated, these critical windows are as sensitive to positive protective factors as they are to stressors, like nutritional deficiency and deprivation.

The actual impact of nutritional inadequacies on the developing brain depend on: the timing and degree of nutrient deficiency, such that, if the deficiency occurs during a time period when the need for that nutrient is high, brain development is most likely to be negatively impacted; a child's experience and inputs from the environment and, lastly, the possibility of recovery through provision of improved conditions [8].

The significant impact of nutritional inadequacies cannot be better exemplified by how stunting, and the interventions implemented to mitigate it, affects children. Stunting, one of the burdens of severe malnutrition, is defined as measuring shorter by more than two standard deviations than the WHO median for their exact age and gender (HAZ) [9]. It is a manifestation of chronic malnutrition in the early years, compromising brain development. Studies worldwide have associated stunting with lower cognitive scores and subsequent academic achievement, but have also observed variables that mitigate its negative impact.

A population-based longitudinal study in Cebu City, Philippines, by Adair et al. [10] found that each standard deviation increase in length for the age Z-score (LAZ) is associated with an additional schooling of 0.40 years, putting an estimate of nearly a full year of total schooling separating the most severely stunted children (LAZ < -3) from those who were not. Catch-up growth from early childhood stunting is vital in cognitive development. This was shown in a large cohort of Peruvian children ($N = 1{,}674$), where it was observed that those who had been stunted before the age of 18 months but were not stunted anymore, upon follow-up at the age of 4–6 years, performed as well in vocabulary and quantitative tests as children who had never been stunted. Meanwhile, significantly lower scores were noted among children who did not experience catch-up growth at all [11]. Similarly, in a cohort study among Vietnamese children, stunting in the first year of life was negatively associated with developmental scores at 2 years of age, but a high-quality home environment appeared to attenuate these associations [12]. These studies show that addressing nutritional conditions, like stunting, in the earliest possible period is imperative because of its positive long-term impact on development, subsequent academic performance, and adult productivity.

Prado and Dewey [13] depicted how a child's physical growth, activity, and overall health influence the way he or she interacts with the environment and eventually how, because of this interaction, the child's motor, cognitive, and socioemotional development proceeds across their life span. These are the scaffolds that should be laid out solidly to harness brain development. The formidability of these scaffolds, however, is tested time and again and calamities like the recent COVID-19 (SARS-CoV-2) global pandemic, and the disruptive systemic ripples that it brought along, has unfortunately shaken these foundations.

Across many low-to-middle income countries, the pandemic heightened household food insecurity, especially among marginalized groups [14, 15]. Food insecurity is defined by the Food and Agriculture Organization as "lacking regular access to enough safe and nutritious food for normal growth and development and an active and healthy life" [16].

In the Philippines, for example, where 1 out of 3 of children less than 5 years old is stunted, mostly attributed by local nutrition experts to suboptimal prenatal conditions and inadequate food security and diversity [17], the pandemic and subsequent lockdown saw a further increase in food-insecure households. A cross-sectional survey done by the Food and Nutrition Research Institute (FNRI) in the last quarter of 2020 showed that 7 out of 10 households, identified to be moderately to severely food insecure, had both a pregnant member and a child/children less than 5 years old. The data further demonstrated that households with children less than 5 years old were 1.3 times more likely to be food insecure [18]. This, of course, does not augur well in the drive to combat stunting and its subsequent adverse effects.

Meanwhile, in some parts of the world, we see the flipside of that problem. Obesity rates were seen to have increased during the pandemic among 2–17-year-old children (average age = 9.2 years) in a large pediatric primary care network in Philadelphia [19]. The study analyzed more than 500,000 visits from January 2019 to December 2020. They noted an increase in the overall obesity prevalence rate from 13.7% in 2019 to 15.4%. Data showed that the highest increase of 2.6% was seen among children aged 5–9 years and underscored that during the pandemic, preexisting disparities in obesity in terms of race and ethnicity, insurance, and neighborhood socioeconomic status widened.

The authors concluded that the rise in the incidence of obesity, especially in children and adolescents during the pandemic, was possibly due to decreased physical activity, stress, overeating, and staying at home almost all the time due to global lockdowns, home isolation, and the closure of schools and online classes.

Even in countries, like Sweden, where there was no formal societal lockdown during the pandemic, obesity rates likewise increased. In a retrospective population-based cross-sectional study that included more than 25,000 3- to 5-

year-olds, increased BMI was seen among 3- to 4-year-olds, more noted among 3-year-old girls. They also noted that children from lower socioeconomic households were at a higher risk for obesity. The authors surmise that the pandemic may have negatively affected health behaviors, even in a less restricted environment [20].

The pandemic also impacted developmental and behavioral concerns among children. Prior to the pandemic, a study by Buenavista-Pacifico et al. [21] noted that the risk for developmental delay among 1- to 2-year-old Filipino children was 11%, but as clinicians were returning to their clinics for face-to-face encounters, the majority of clinicians informally surveyed in a Philippine private tertiary hospital noted an average of 2–4 out of 10 children aged 1–3 years old having concerns regarding developmental surveillance. Speech and language delay was the most significant concern followed by social and interactive skills. Other concerns revolved around the unregulated use of gadgets, sleep, and feeding issues.

Similar findings were also demonstrated in an unpublished descriptive cross-sectional study by Caballas et al. among 12- to 36-month-olds seen in a private tertiary hospital. The authors noted that 1 out of 4 or 25% of 1- to 3-year-olds included in the study were at risk for developmental delays with a two-fold increased risk for children with more than an hour of screen time.

Further effects of increased screen time during the pandemic were shown in a study out of Australia among preschool children [22]. All of the children in the study were exposed to online content with the duration ranging from 1 to 2 h. A greater screen time was associated with a shorter sleep duration, predicted lower communication and problem-solving scores, along with more attention difficulties.

These observations were not only noted among toddlers and young children during the pandemic, but similar effects were also seen on early neurodevelopment among infants.

The COMBO study or the COVID-19 Mother Baby Outcomes Initiative from Columbia University looked at the association of birth during the COVID-19 pandemic with the neurodevelopmental status at 6 months in infants with or without in-utero exposure to maternal COVID-19 infection [23]. The Ages and Stages Questionnaire (ASQ)-3 was used to assess neurodevelopmental domains among subjects. The findings of this cohort study of 255 infants suggest that exposure to maternal infection in utero was not associated with differences in neurodevelopmental scores. However, what was unsettling was the finding that both exposed and unexposed infants born during the height of the pandemic from March to December 2020 had significantly lower scores on gross motor, fine motor, and personal–social subdomains compared with a historical cohort of infants born before the onset of the pandemic.

Parallel to this, another study also aimed to characterize cognitive function in young children less than 3 years of age over the past decade and to test whether children exhibit different cognitive development profiles through the COVID-19 pandemic. Using the Mullen Scales of Early Learning (MSEL), researchers from the Resonance Consortium study examined the general cognitive scores of 700 healthy and neurotypically developing children in 2020 and 2021 and compared these to the preceding decade, 2011–2019 [24]. Like the COMBO study, what they found was that children born during the pandemic, even in the absence of a direct SARS-CoV-2 infection and COVID-19 illness, have significantly reduced verbal, motor, and overall cognitive performance compared to the children born prepandemic, with males and children in lower socioeconomic families being the most affected.

These findings are further supported by another study (LENA Foundation) that looked at speech and language behavior and development among COVID-era children or those who were born within December 2020. The vocalizations and conversational turns of these children were compared to their pre-COVID peers. The results showed that children from the COVID-era sample scored lower across all measurements than their pre-COVID peers, experiencing fewer conversational turns, hearing fewer adult words, and producing fewer vocalizations [25].

These results highlight that the environmental changes associated with the COVID-19 pandemic may have significantly and negatively affected infant and child behavior and development.

Conclusion

The early years of life are inarguably the most sensitive periods of a child's development and learning. Positive factors protect this epoch but toxic stressors, like the global pandemic and lockdown, have buffeted the scaffolds of early brain development from the perspective of nutrition and environmental stimulation. As we pivot after the pandemic, modifiable factors, like nutrition, social interaction, and developmental stimulation, need to be revisited, protected, and enriched more than ever.

There is a renewed call for pediatricians and other healthcare practitioners in clinics and communities globally to more ardently screen, monitor for, and provide proper advice for concerns in growth and development during the first 3 years of life to help mitigate the impact of the current global events on children's potential to adapt, learn, and be productive adults in the future. Healthcare practitioners should not only act as good counsel for parents in terms of adequate, appropriate, and timely nutrition across their lifespan, beginning from conception, but also as champions for the basic rights of children to a safe, secure, and nurturing environment. Lastly, proactive promotion and protection of social interactions in language-enriched home, school, and community milieus should also be instituted. In the best of worlds, we hope that with early, responsive, and actionable programs, no child will truly be left behind.

Conflict of Interest Statement

Dr. Benitez is a member of the advisory panel of Wyeth Nutrition and a member of the speakers' bureau and key opinion leaders' panel of Wyeth Nutrition Philippines.

Funding Sources

The author received lecture honoraria and travel reimbursement from Nestlé Nutrition Institute.

References

1 Center on the Developing Child Harvard University. Brain Architecture [cited 2023 Aug 12]. Available from: https://developingchild.harvard.edu/science/key-concepts/brain-architecture/.

2 Shonkoff JP, Phillips DA. The developing brain. In: From Neurons to Neighborhoods: The Science of Early Childhood Development. National Academies Press (US), 2000 [cited 2023 Aug 15]. Available from: https://www.ncbi.nlm.nih.gov/books/NBK225562/.

3 Silbereis JC, Pochareddy S, Zhu Y, Li M, Sestan N. The cellular and molecular landscapes of the developing human central nervous system. Neuron. 2016;89(2):248–68. https://doi.org/10.1016/j.neuron.2015.12.008.

4 Lake A, Chan M. Putting science into practice for early child development. Lancet. 2015;385(9980):1816–7. https://doi.org/10.1016/S0140-6736(14)61680-9.

5 Pujol J, Soriano-Mas C, Ortiz H, Sebastian-Galles N, Losilla JM, Deus J. Myelination of language-related areas in the developing brain. Neurology. 2006;66(3):339–43. https://doi.org/10.1212/01.wnl.0000201049.66073.8d.

6 Deoni SCL,Dean D, Joelson S, O'Regan J, Schneider N. Early nutrition influences developmental myelination and cognition in infants and young children. Neuroimage. 2018;178:649–59. https://doi.org/10.1016/j.neuroimage.2017.12.056.

7 Schneider N, Bruchhage MMK, O'Neill B, Hartweg M, Tanguy J, Steiner P, et al. A nutrient formulation affects developmental myelination in term infants: a randomized clinical trial. Front Nutr. 2022;9:823893. https://doi.org/10.3389/fnut.2022.823893.

8 Prado EI, Dewey KG. Nutrition and brain development in early life. Nutr Rev. 2014;72(4):267–84. https://doi.org/10.1111/nure.12102.

9 World Health Organization. Stunting in A Nutshell [cited 2023 Aug 15]. Available from: https://www.who.int/news/item/19-11-2015-stunting-in-a-nutshell.

10 Adair LS, Carba DB, Lee NR, Boria JB. Stunting, IQ and final school attainment in the Cebu longitudinal health and nutrition survey birth cohort. Econ Hum Biol. 2021;42:100999. https://doi.org/10.1016/j.ehb.2021.100999.

11 Crookston BT, Penny ME, Alder SC, Dickerson TT, Merrill RM, Stanford JB, et al. Children who recover from early stunting and children who are not stunted demonstrate similar levels of cognition. J Nutr. 2010;140(11):1996–2001. https://doi.org/10.3945/jn.109.118927.

12 Nguyen PH, DiGirolamo AM, Gonzalez-Casanova I, Young M, Kim N, Nguyen S, et al. Influences of early child nutritional status and home learning environment on child development in Vietnam. Matern Child Nutr. 2018;14(1):e12468. https://doi.org/10.1111/mcn.12468.

13 Prado EI, Dewey KG. Nutrition and brain development in early life. Nutr Rev. 2014;72(4):267–84. https://doi.org/10.1111/nure.12102.
14 HongZhu P, Mhango SN, Vinnakota A, Mansour M, Coss-Bu A. Effects of COVID-19 pandemic on nutritional status, feeding practices, and access to food among infants and children in lower and middle-income countries: a narrative review. Curr Trop Med Rep. 2022;9(4):197–206. https://doi.org/10.1007/s40475-022-00271-8.
15 Karim KMR, Tasnim T. Impact of lockdown due to COVID-19 on nutrition and food security of the selected low-income households in Bangladesh. Heliyon. 2022;8(5):e09368. https://doi.org/10.1016/j.heliyon.2022.e09368.
16 Food and Agriculture Organization of the United States. Hunger and Food Insecurity. [cited 2023 Aug 10]. Available from: https://www.fao.org/hunger/en/
17 Capanzana MV, Demombynes G, Gubbins P. Why are so many children stunted in the Philippines? World Bank Policy Research Working Paper 9294 on Health Nutrition and Population. 2020 [cited 2023 Aug 10]. Available from: https://thedocs.worldbank.org/en/doc/823021598886801368009002 2020/original/TF0A8125WhyAreSoManyChildrenStuntedinthePhilippines.pdf.
18 Angeles-Agdeppa I, Javier CA, Duante CA, Maniego MLV. Impacts of COVID-19 pandemic on household food security and access to social protection programs in the Philippines: findings from a telephone rapid nutrition assessment survey. Food Nutr Bull. 2022;43(2):213–31. https://doi.org/10.1177/03795721221078363.
19 Jenssen BP, Kelly MK, Powell M, Bouchelle Z, Mayne SL, Fiks AG. COVID-19 and changes in child obesity. Pediatrics. 2021;147(5):e2021050123. https://doi.org/10.1542/peds.2021-050123.
20 Faldt A, Nejat S, Sollander S, Durbeej N, Holmgren A. Increased incidence of overweight and obesity among preschool Swedish children during the COVID-19 pandemic. Eur J Public Health. 2023;33(1):127–31. https://doi.org/10.1093/eurpub/ckac181.
21 Buenavista-Pacifico MR, Reyes AL, Benitez BC, Villanueva-Uy E, Lam HY, Ostrea JEM. The prevalence of developmental delay among Filipino children at ages 6, 12 and 24 months based on the griffiths mental development scales. Acta Med Philipp. 2018;52(6). https://doi.org/10.47895/amp.v52i6.277.
22 Axelsson EL, Purcell K, Asis A, Paech G, Metse A, Murphy D, et al. Preschoolers' engagement with screen content and associations with sleep and cognitive development. Acta Psychol. 2022;230:103762. https://doi.org/10.1016/j.actpsy.2022.103762.
23 Shuffrey LC, Firestein MR,Kyle MH, Fields A, Alcantara C, Dima A, et al. Association of birth during the COVID-19 pandemic with neurodevelopmental status at 6 months in infants with and without in utero exposure to maternal SARS-CoV-2 infection. JAMA Pediatr. 2022;176(6):e215563. https://doi.org/10.1001/jamapediatrics.2021.5563.
24 Deoni SCL, Beauchemin J, Volpe A, D'Sa V, the Resonance Consortium. Impact of the COVID-19 pandemic on early child cognitive development: initial findings in a longitudinal observational study of child health. MedRxiv(pre-print). 2021. https://doi.org/10.1101/2021.08.10.21261846.
25 LENA Team. COVID-Era Infants Vocalize Less and Experience Fewer Conversational Turns [cited 2023 Aug 10]. Available from: https://www.lena.org/covid-infant-vocalizations-conversational-turns/

Bernadette C. Benitez
Section of Developmental and Behavioral Pediatrics, Department of Pediatrics
Makati Medical Center
2 Amorsolo Street
Makati City 1209, Metro Manila, Philippines
bicbenitez@yahoo.com

Published online: November 15, 2024

Szajewska H, Neu J, Shamir R, Wong G, Prentice AM (eds): Shaping the Future with Nutrition. Nestle Nutr Inst Workshop Ser. Basel, Karger, 2024, vol 100, pp 90–99 (DOI: 10.1159/000540142)

The Art of Chewing: Optimizing Early Life Sensory Exposure to Develop Healthy Eating Behavior

Marlou P. Lasschuijt Ciarán G. Forde

Sensory Science and Eating Behaviour Group, Division of Human Nutrition and Health, Wageningen University and Research, Wageningen, The Netherlands

Abstract

Eating behavior and food preferences are shaped in early life and contribute to lifelong food choices. Much of the current dietary advice for infants and toddlers focuses on the nutritional quality of foods, with less emphasis on food sensory qualities. However, exposure to age-appropriate sensory properties, such as tastes and textures, are key in shaping early-life eating behaviors and food preferences. During weaning, new-borns rely on reflexes such as sucking and rooting to get sufficient nutrient intake. Around 6 months of age infants transit from dependent feeding with liquid foods such as breast or bottle feeding, to independent feeding with solid foods. During this rapid learning period, the infant must learn to sit upright and balance their head and quickly develop in terms of oral anatomy, emerging of teeth as well as the muscle coordination needed to orally process food. Different product textures require unique oral processing skills that have to be acquired through experience with food oral breakdown and swallowing. These early food experiences shape the eating behaviors that become habitual and are carried forward into later childhood. Early life feeding strategies vary widely across populations but become all the more challenging in specific child populations such as children who received early life tube-feeding and children with developmental challenges are further complicated by anatomical issues and acquired negative associations with food. Due to the significance of early life food sensory exposure in shaping dietary behavior, there is a need for science-based recommendations to help guide this sensory learning to inform dietary behaviors in both healthy and clinical child populations.

Introduction

Eating behavior and dietary habits developed in early life play an important role in shaping subsequent healthy dietary patterns [1]. During the early childhood years, the emphasis is often on the nutritional quality of complementary foods, including the provision of foods from each food group according to dietary guidelines to ensure essential nutrient intake necessary for growth and development [2]. However, less emphasis is given to the importance of food sensory properties exposure during early life, such as tastes and textures, which are key in shaping food acceptance and healthy dietary behaviors (see Fig. 1).

Taste and Texture are important sensory aspects of food that determine food acceptance and this has been extensively researched in children [3]. We know that infants exhibit an innate preference for sweet, and an innate dislike for bitter tastes as these tastes inherently signal energy (glucose needed for the developing brain) and toxicity, respectively [4]. These preferences emerge as early as 32 weeks gestation and are further shaped by the taste profile of the foods consumed by the mother [5]. The experiential learning of flavor preferences continues through sensory exposure to tastes and flavors in breastmilk or infant formula, and through food exposure during the complementary feeding period [4]. Throughout toddlerhood, food preferences are then further shaped by the influence of many factors including being exposed to a wide variety of different foods, family meal practices, and the social environment [6].

Childrens' preferences and aversions for specific sensory aspects of food significantly impacts *what* they consume and *how* they consume it, and these behaviors can affect the way they eat and amount of food consumed [7]. How food is consumed, in terms of oral processing, is determined by how the infant

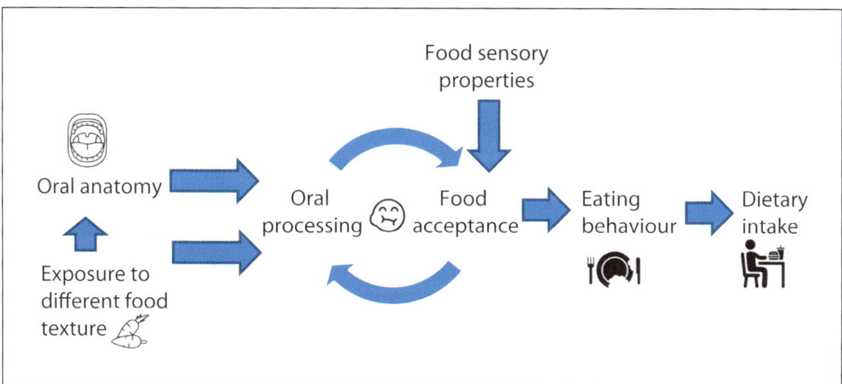

Fig. 1. The process of developing dietary behavior in early life.

interprets the structural properties of these foods, alongside the emergence of their eating behavior phenotype [8]. When infants have a higher eating rate combined with foods that can be consumed at a more rapid eating rate, this leads to a larger meal size and higher energy intake. Faster consumption can promote habitual excess calorie intake before the body signals fullness and potentially leads to sustained positive energy balance and an increased risk of overweight and obesity [9]. Conversely, developmental challenges that make it difficult to orally process food may lead to disruptions in learning fullness and hunger signals or a dislike of foods with challenging texture properties. This in turn may lead to inadequate nutrient and energy intakes and potentially hinder growth and development in early life.

Combined, early sensory exposure and the development of eating behaviors play a key role in determining the type of foods selected and the amount in which they are consumed. This chapter provides an overview of eating behavior development and how it relates to food preferences and dietary patterns in healthy and specific (clinical) child populations.

Eating Behavior Development

Newborns rely on their innate sucking, swallowing, and rooting reflexes to consume breast milk or infant formula milk. Their tongue movements are limited to protrusion to push food in or out, and the tongue is held in place by fat deposits in the cheeks, which also helps to form a vacuum for stronger suction. This limited movement also helps reduce the risk of swallowing the tongue during feeding. In the subsequent post-partum months, the infants, oral anatomy develops rapidly, alongside the ability to coordinate oral-facial muscles. Around 6 months of age, the infants, oral cavity has changed significantly with the loss of fat deposits in the cheeks to create more space in the oral cavity to allow for rotary movements of the tongue. The palate doubles in width, length, and height to allow for healthy tooth eruption as the infant experiences more solid textures for the first time. Exposure to textures during this period has a synergistic effect of encouraging the lengthening of the palate and the emergence of straight dentition, to better equip the infant for chewing, while also providing opportunities for experiential learning to further develop chewing skills. These anatomical changes enable the infant to transit from liquids to semi-solids, soft solids, and finally to foods with a more challenging harder texture. During the toddler years (1–3 years), children gain better control over their tongue movements, allowing them to move their tongue laterally and in circular motions to move food particles between their molars for more efficient crushing. This is a complex fine motor skill that involves the coordination of 26 muscle pairs and is controlled by five cranial nerves. Unlike sweet taste preferences, we are not born with any innate ability to know "how to eat", and this complex ballet of synchronized contraction and relaxation has to be learned through the infants experience and interaction with novel food textures, all while trying to sustain adequate energy intakes and avoiding the constant risk of choking [10].

Early life experiences with food may have a lasting impact on oral anatomy, oral processing behavior, and, ultimately on food preferences and dietary patterns. Once toddlers develop these oral processing skills, they tend to remain stable throughout later childhood. Oral processing behavior can be considered a strong personal trait, such that when the same food is consumed the person will show similar oral processing behaviors over time. There is considerable variation in oral processing behaviors between people, yet these behaviors appear to remain stable over time and can play a significant role in habitual energy intakes within meals, over time. Oral processing also sets the rate at which a food can be eaten which is dependent on both the eating rate of the individual and the structural challenge posed by the food being consumed. Research in children and adults has shown that a "fast-eating" phenotype characterized by larger bite sizes, and little chewing per bite, combined with a preference for softly textured energy-dense foods, are associated with higher habitual energy intakes compared to those with slower eating phenotypes with a preference for hard textured foods [11, 12]. Research has shown that toddlers who were observed to have a faster eating rate were still classified as eating faster 3 years later, and had a more rapid weight gain and adiposity levels compared to those with a relatively slower eating rate [13]. Little is known about the extent to which early-age feeding practices can shape these habitual oral processing behaviors and eating styles. While there is evidence to suggest that breastfeeding can influence feeding voracity and oral anatomy, offering protection against malocclusions, posterior crossbites, and teeth crowding, there is limited evidence to show this influence extends further to influence a child's oral processing behavior or eating rate. A critical period in early life that may shape longer-term dietary behavior is the complementary feeding phase.

Texture Introduction during Complementary Feeding

Complementary feeding is the introduction of semi-solid and solid foods alongside breast milk or formula and is a sensitive period in shaping food preferences and eating behavior. However, there is a general lack of consistency in the guidelines for best practices for caregivers on *how* and *when* to introduce new foods with more complex food textures to their child. This is further complicated by differences among infants and toddlers of the same age in terms of oral development and oral processing skills creating a discrepancy between chronological age and developmental readiness to consume foods with more complex and challenging textures.

A French survey of >3,000 mothers revealed a wide variation in feeding practices regarding the introduction of complementary foods. Mothers often rely on cues from their children to indicate when to transition to more complex textures, for example when their child had more teeth or demonstrated the ability to hold a spoon or food in their hands. However, researchers found that the number of teeth did not affect the ability to break down a gel given in a mesh-feeder and although older infants performed better in the oral-break-down of food there were significant variations between children of the same age. This might have been due to differences in early-life experience with oral processing of different types of food texture. Therefore, neither age nor number of teeth were direct predictors of determining the texture readiness of a child, as this is better predicted by the child's developmental stage and experience with a wide variety of more diverse and challenging textures [14]. When introducing novel foods to infants or toddlers it is important to consider its textural properties and associated oral processing techniques needed for a safe swallow of a food bolus. For example, harder pieces that are difficult to squeeze into smaller particles with jaws or the tongue against the palate are not suited for young infants, and foods with soft-airy textures such as bread may pose a risk, as these food particles can easily be breathed or sucked into the airways. Adding margarine or another lubricant to bread may reduce this risk. Foods with multiple layers of texture or foods that fragment into many smaller hard particles can often pose a challenge to the child's nascent oral processing skills, where tongue movements and mouth clearance are not fully developed. Conversely, foods that are easily formed into a pasty bolus such as soft crackers or baby corn puffs/sticks can be given at an earlier developmental stage. Early-life exposure to different food textures promote oral processing skills and this has been linked to acceptance of a broader range of foods [10]. For example, toddlers, who have developed more advanced chewing skills tend to exhibit higher acceptance for more complex textured foods, such as baby biscuits compared to younger infants [15]. Research has shown that infants exposed to a wider variety of textures consumed larger portions of chopped carrots compared to those with less food texture experience at 12 months [16]. Studies show that food preference reflects early exposure and experience with food textures and its relationship with the ability to orally process foods [15].

Eating Behavior Development in Clinical or Atypically Developing Child Populations

Much of our understanding of the development of early-life feeding strategies derives from research in specific child (clinical) populations. For example, children or infants whose first experience with food has been through tube feeding are prone to develop eating behavior problems when transitioning from breast milk or formula to solid foods. Another population in which eating behavior problems arise are children with oral-facial development challenges such as those common in Children with Downs syndrome.

Eating Behavior Development of Infants Who Received Tube Feeding

Energy intake of hospitalized (pre-term) infants is often low due to issues such as difficulty with coordination of sucking movements, fatigue, or because of higher energy requirements due to illness or to prepare an infant for surgery [17]. When energy intake of hospitalized infants is insufficient for a longer period of time, many receive tube feeding. Tube feeding is common in pre-term born infants as they often do not yet have the neurological or digestive maturation to process oral ingestion of breast milk or formula. Infants who receive tube feeding during the first months, or years, of their life are at a higher risk to develop appetite dysregulation issues, hypersensitivity to food sensory properties, and food avoidance behavior [18].

Infants who receive long-term tube feeding may develop impaired satiety responses when the timing of feeding is discordant with the infants' appetite [19]. To prevent negative health outcomes associated with scheduled feeding, infants can be fed based on their appetite cues. Cue-based feeding helps the infant to regulate their food intake by responding to their internal appetite feelings and longer term this may lead to better satiety responsiveness and longer-term healthy body weight development [20].

Besides cue-based feeding, oral stimulation during tube feeding can improve oral-facial muscle coordination required for sucking and swallowing and helps entrain the oral processing needed for transition to solid foods post-tube feeding. For example, non-nutritive sucking on pacifiers has been shown to improve coordination of sucking movements of infants, supporting the transition to bottle feeding, and has been associated with shorter hospital stay and reduced stress levels [21]. Contrary, a lack of or limited oral stimulation during the first months of life may lead to hypersensitivity to tactile stimuli such as food textures [18]. Dislike for specific textures in infants who have received tube feeding may be due to the limited exposure to textures during the complementary feeding phase which may lead to reduced experiential learning and difficulty with oral processing specific textures that may not have been developed due to their inexperience [22]. There are several tools that can be used by medical professionals to assess whether infants can receive oral nutrition or oral-feeding readiness such as the Oral Feeding Readiness scale, and neonatal oral-motor-assessment scale [23].

In more severe cases, transitioning from tube-feeding to normal eating behaviors may induce strong food avoidance which leads to persistent tube-feeding. One study showed that 70% of pre-term infants that were tube-fed in the ICU are still tube-dependent 6 months after their hospital discharge [24]. The transition from tube to oral feeding in these children can be made more successful by using the "hunger provocation method", which requires the child to signal hunger and feed on demand rather than on a schedule, and has been shown to be successful in >80% of children compared to only 10% who successfully transition from tube to oral feeding [25].

Eating Behavior Development of Children with Down Syndrome

Children with Down Syndrome (CWDS) can have a typical oral-facial anatomy that may lead to difficulties with oral processing of food. These oral-facial characteristics include macroglossia, poor occlusal contacts, and hypotonic oro-facial muscle development and coordination [26]. These characteristics often lead to difficulties in consuming foods, initially starting with breastfeeding where issues arise due to poor lip-seal, slow sucking, and a perceived increased risk of choking and aspiration. As such, breastfeeding rates tend to be much lower among CWDS compared to other children, although research shows most CWDS can be successfully breastfed if mothers receive the right support. Breastfeeding of CWDS is especially important as this promotes oral muscle coordination, shaping of the oral cavity, and speech development [27].

The transition from breast or bottle feeding to solid foods is delayed in CWDS compared to other child populations. For example, the introduction of bread is delayed by 4 months compared to peers [28]. This creates a cycle that hinders the longer-term development of oral processing and texture learning early in life. These delays are associated with impaired oral function, lower texture acceptance, and difficulties in consuming solid foods, potentially leading to picky eating and increased risks of choking and aspiration [29]. Because of this, CWDS may develop a preference for foods that do not require oral processing or to use sucking movements as much as possible. Additionally, parents are inclined to give their child foods with a semi-solid or soft solid texture [30]. This shapes a preference for foods that can be consumed easily and with a fast eating rate. These types of foods generally have low satiating capacity and are therefore often overconsumed. If these preference for easy-to-consume foods persist into adulthood this may shape dietary behavior that increases the risk of overweight or obesity [31].

Conclusion

Early life food sensory exposure affects food familiarity, food preferences, and oral processing skill. Combined these factors affect the development of healthy dietary patterns. Evidence from research in specific (clinical) child populations has shown that early behavioral nutrition interventions can significantly enhance eating behaviors. Despite the important role of sensory exposure in shaping dietary patterns, there are limited guidelines for parents or health care professionals on how to introduce taste and texture to the diet of infants or toddlers. There is thus a need for science-based sensory recommendations to help shape healthy dietary behaviors tailored to specific clinical child populations.

Conflict of Interest Statement

The authors have no conflicts of interest to declare in relation to the current manuscript.

Funding Sources

M.P.L. received lecture honoraria and travel reimbursement from Nestlé Nutrition Institute.

The authors have received the following research funding relevant to the topic of the current manuscript, but outcomes or data of these research projects are not included in the current manuscript:

Technology development to measure breastmilk intake – Flow project, funding sources: seed grants EWUU and 4TU NIRICT program.

Cue-based feeding in NICU infants – Eat Sleep Research Repeat project, funding source: seed grant EWUU.

Research related to eating rate and food texture – Restructure project, funding source: Dutch Top-Consortium for Knowledge and Innovation Agri & Food (TKI-Agri-food) Project Restructure; (TKI 22.150).

Author Contributions

C.G.F. and M.P.L. developed the outline and wrote the manuscript.

References

1 Koletzko B, von Kries R, Monasterolo RC, Subias JE, Scaglioni S, Giovannini M, et al, eds. Infant Feeding and Later Obesity Risk. Early Nutrition Programming and Health Outcomes in Later Life. Dordrecht: Springer Netherlands; 2009.

2 Corrêa Rezende JL, de Medeiros Frazão Duarte MC, Melo GRDAE, Santos LCd, Toral N. Food-based dietary guidelines for children and adolescents. Front Public Health. 2022;10:1033580. https://doi.org/10.3389/fpubh.2022.1033580

3 McCrickerd K, Forde CG. Sensory influences on food intake control: moving beyond palatability. Obes Rev. 2016;17(1):18–29. https://doi.org/10.1111/obr.12340

4 Ventura AK, Worobey J. Early influences on the development of food preferences. Curr Biol. 2013; 23(9):R401–8. https://doi.org/10.1016/j.cub.2013.02.037

5 Ustun B, Reissland N, Covey J, Schaal B, Blissett J. Flavor sensing in utero and emerging discriminative behaviors in the human fetus. Psychol Sci. 2022;33(10):1651–63. https://doi.org/10.1177/09567976221105460

6 Mennella JA. Development of food preferences: lessons learned from longitudinal and experimental studies. Food Qual Prefer. 2006;17(7-8): 635–7. https://doi.org/10.1016/j.foodqual.2006.01.008

7 Forde CG. From perception to ingestion; the role of sensory properties in energy selection, eating behaviour and food intake. Food Qual Prefer. 2018; 66:171–7. https://doi.org/10.1016/j.foodqual.2018.01.010

8 Bolhuis DP, Forde CG. Application of food texture to moderate oral processing behaviors and energy intake. Trends Food Sci Technol. 2020;106:445–56. https://doi.org/10.1016/j.tifs.2020.10.021

9 Lasschuijt MP, de Graaf K, Mars M. Effects of oro-sensory exposure on satiation and underlying neurophysiological mechanisms—what do we know so far? Nutrients. 2021;13(5):1391. https://doi.org/10.3390/nu13051391

10 Tournier C, Forde CG. Food oral processing and eating behavior from infancy to childhood: evidence on the role of food texture in the development of healthy eating behavior. Crit Rev Food Sci Nutr. 2023:1–14. https://doi.org/10.1080/10408398.2023.2214227

11 Robinson E, Almiron-Roig E, Rutters F, de Graaf C, Forde CG, Tudur Smith C, et al. A systematic review and meta-analysis examining the effect of eating rate on energy intake and hunger. Am J Clin Nutr. 2014;100(1):123–51. https://doi.org/10.3945/ajcn.113.081745

12 Janani R, Tan VWK, Goh AT, Choy MJY, Lim AJ, Teo PS, et al. Independent and combined impact of texture manipulation on oral processing behaviours among faster and slower eaters. Food Funct. 2022;13(18):9340–54. https://doi.org/10.1039/d2fo00485b

13 Fogel A, Goh AT, Fries LR, Sadananthan SA, Velan SS, Michael N, et al. A description of an 'obesogenic' eating style that promotes higher energy intake and is associated with greater adiposity in 4.5 year-old children: results from the GUSTO cohort. Physiol Behav. 2017;176:107–16. https://doi.org/10.1016/j.physbeh.2017.02.013

14 Tournier C, Demonteil L, Canon F, Marduel A, Feron G, Nicklaus S. A new masticatory performance assessment method for infants: a feasibility study. J Texture Stud. 2019;50(3):237–47. https://doi.org/10.1111/jtxs.12388

15 Demonteil L, Tournier C, Marduel A, Dusoulier M, Weenen H, Nicklaus S. Longitudinal study on acceptance of food textures between 6 and 18 months. Food Qual Prefer. 2019;71:54–65. https://doi.org/10.1016/j.foodqual.2018.05.010

16 Blossfeld I, Collins A, Kiely M, Delahunty C. Texture preferences of 12-month-old infants and the role of early experiences. Food Qual Prefer. 2007;18(2):396–404. https://doi.org/10.1016/j.foodqual.2006.03.022

17 Gottrand F, Sullivan PB. Gastrostomy tube feeding: when to start, what to feed and how to stop. Eur J Clin Nutr. 2010;64(suppl 1):S17–21. https://doi.org/10.1038/ejcn.2010.43

18 Mason SJ, Harris G, Blissett J. Tube feeding in infancy: implications for the developmentof normal eating and drinking skills. Dysphagia. 2005; 20(1):46–61. https://doi.org/10.1007/s00455-004-0025-2

19 Mason SJ, Harris G, Blissett J. Tube feeding in infancy: implications for the development of normal eating and drinking skills. Dysphagia. 2005;20(1):46–61. https://doi.org/10.1007/s00455-004-0025-2

20 Shaker CS. Cue-based feeding in the NICU: using the infant's communication as a guide. Neonatal Netw. 2013;32(6):404–8. https://doi.org/10.1891/0730-0832.32.6.404

21 Pinelli J, Symington A. Non-nutritive sucking for promoting physiologic stability and nutrition in preterm infants. Cochrane Database Syst Rev. 2005;4:CD001071. https://doi.org/10.1002/14651858.CD001071.pub2
22 Gisel EG. Effect of food texture on the development of chewing of children between six months and two years of age. Dev Med Child Neurol. 1991;33(1):69–79. https://doi.org/10.1111/j.1469-8749.1991.tb14786.x
23 Bickell M, Barton C, Dow K, Fucile S. A systematic review of clinical and psychometric properties of infant oral motor feeding assessments. Dev Neurorehabil. 2018;21(6):351–61. https://doi.org/10.1080/17518423.2017.1289272
24 Williams SL, Popowics NM, Tadesse DG, Poindexter BB, Merhar SL. Tube feeding outcomes of infants in a Level IV NICU. J Perinatol. 2019;39(10):1406–10. https://doi.org/10.1038/s41372-019-0449-z
25 Clouzeau H, Dipasquale V, Rivard L, Lecoeur K, Lecoufle A, Le Ru-Raguénès V, et al. Weaning children from prolonged enteral nutrition: a position paper. Eur J Clin Nutr. 2022;76(4):505–15. https://doi.org/10.1038/s41430-021-00992-5
26 Cañizares-Prado S, Molina-López J, Moya MT, Planells E. Oral function and eating habit problems in people with Down syndrome. Int J Environ Res Public Health. 2022;19(5):2616. https://doi.org/10.3390/ijerph19052616
27 Jonsson L, Olsson Tyby C, Hullfors S, Lundqvist P. Mothers of children with down syndrome: a qualitative study of experiences of breastfeeding and breastfeeding support. Scand J Caring Sci. 2022;36(4):1156–64. https://doi.org/10.1111/scs.13088
28 Hopman E, Csizmadia CG, Bastiani WF, Engels QM, De Graaf EA, Le Cessie S, et al. Eating habits of young children with Down syndrome in The Netherlands: adequate nutrient intakes but delayed introduction of solid food. J Am Diet Assoc. 1998;98(7):790–4. https://doi.org/10.1016/s0002-8223(98)00178-3
29 Roccatello G, Cocchi G, Dimastromatteo RT, Cavallo A, Biserni GB, Selicati M, et al. Eating and lifestyle habits in youth with Down syndrome attending a care program: an exploratory lesson for future improvements. Front Nutr. 2021;8:641112. https://doi.org/10.3389/fnut.2021.641112
30 Ross CF, Bernhard CB, Surette V, Hasted A, Wakeling I, Smith-Simpson S. Eating behaviors in children with Down syndrome: results of a home-use test. J Texture Stud. 2022;53(5):629–46. https://doi.org/10.1111/jtxs.12703
31 Ross CF, Bernhard CB, Smith-Simpson S. Parent-reported ease of eating foods of different textures in young children with Down syndrome. J Texture Stud. 2019;50(5):426–33. https://doi.org/10.1111/jtxs.12410

Marlou P. Lasschuijt
Sensory Science and Eating Behaviour Group
Division of Human Nutrition and Health
Wageningen University & Research
Stippeneng 4
6708 WE Wageningen, The Netherlands
marlou.lasschuijt@wur.nl

Published online: November 15, 2024

Szajewska H, Neu J, Shamir R, Wong G, Prentice AM (eds): Shaping the Future with Nutrition. Nestle Nutr Inst Workshop Ser. Basel, Karger, 2024, vol 100, pp 100–110 (DOI: 10.1159/000540211)

Strategies to Develop Balanced Dietary Habits: Solving the Dilemma

Eslam Tawfik ElBaroudy[a, b]

[a]Department of Pediatrics, Sheikh Khalifa Medical City, Abu Dhabi, UAE; [b]Department of Pediatrics, Faculty of Medicine, Suez University, Suez, Egypt

Abstract

Micronutrient deficiencies in children can occur for multiple reasons, including poor access to food, particular dietary patterns or health conditions that may impact nutrient absorption and utilization. Reduced access to food for infants and young children can lead to malnutrition, increasing the risk of infectious diseases, poor growth, cognitive impairment, emotional dysfunction, and even death. Due to the limited foods available, children with malnutrition also often experience low micronutrient intake. Selective or picky eating is a common feeding difficulty in young children worldwide and can have adverse effects on health and development. Selective eaters generally consume a less diverse diet, leading to an imbalanced nutrient intake. Dietary supplementation provides an individually targeted approach to address micronutrient deficiencies. This strategy has been used safely and effectively to prevent micronutrient deficiencies in high-income countries for over a century. It is the mandatory or voluntary addition of essential micronutrients to widely consumed staple foods and condiments during production. However, worldwide data suggest low compliance with dietary supplementation approaches. This leaves a question mark over the effectiveness of commercial food fortification and highlights the need for improved infrastructure to ensure food fortification or micronutrient supplementation in areas where there is an increased risk of deficiencies.

Introduction

The World Health Organization (WHO) estimates that more than 2 billion people worldwide are deficient in micronutrients such as iron, iodine, zinc, and vitamin A [1]. One-third of these are children under 5 years old, with the majority of malnourished children living in developing countries such as India [2]. In India, over 6,000 children under the age of 5 die every day, with over half of these deaths being attributed to diseases caused by micronutrient deficiency (MND), mainly due to the deficiency of Vitamin A, iron, iodine, and folic acid.

MND-related diseases are responsible for causing high rates of morbidity and mortality in children, particularly those under the age of 5; for example, approximately 0.33 million child deaths every year are caused by vitamin A deficiency in India [3].

There are multiple underlying causes for micronutrient deficiencies, with the most common being related to an imbalanced diet pattern. This can lead to inadequate intake of a wide variety of foods, which would normally each contain a different combination of macro and micronutrients to meet nutritional needs. Poor diet diversity may be associated with limited access to food and malnutrition, certain dietary patterns, or dietary preferences, such as those seen with selective eating behaviors.

Selective Eating

Selective eating, also known as picky eating, is often considered a mild form of feeding difficulty, with more severe eating disorders, such as those related to autism spectrum disorders, at the other end of the spectrum [4].

Although a formal definition of picky eating is not agreed upon, it typically includes the refusal or restriction of familiar and unfamiliar foods, often indicating a sort of neophobia [5]. Selective eating is frequently observed in young children and can result in significant parental stress and negatively affect family relationships [6]. The issue is usually resolved with little or no medical intervention [7].

Feeding difficulties such as picky eating are primarily observed in developed countries where there is more scope for food selection and encompass a complicated set of interactions between parents/caregivers and children, focusing on selecting and consuming food [5].

Several methods evaluate picky eating, leading to significant variation within reported prevalence rates, as stated in Table 1 [7]. Picky eating may be due to

Table 1. Prevalence of picky eating in different countries

Authors	Country	Age (years)	Prevalence (%)	Assessment method
Xue et al. (2015) [11]	China	7–12	59.3	Single item
Xue, Zhao, et al. (2015)	China	3–7	54.0	Single item
Cardona Cano et al. (2015) [13]	The Netherlands	1.5 3 6	26.5 27.6 13.2	CBCL – 2 items
Haszard et al. (2014)	New Zealand	4–8	36.5	LBC – 5 items
Jani Mehta et al. (2014)	Australia	1–5	34.1	Single item
Li et al. (2014)	China	25–36 months	36.2	Study-specific questionnaire
Tharner et al. (2014) [10]	The Netherlands	4	5.6	CEBQ – latent profile approach – 6 items
Horst et al. (2014)	USA	3–4	15.6	Several items
Akamatsu et al. (2013)	Japan	1.5	12.7–38.7	Several items
Hafstad et al. (2013)	Norway	1.5–4.5	22–35	Two items
Finistrella et al. (2012)	Italy	1	20	CFQ – 3 items
Orun et al. (2012)	Turkey	12–72 months	Overall 39	Single item
Goh and Jacob (2012) [6]	Singapore	1–10	40.8	Single item
Micali et al. (2011)	Denmark	5–7	7.3	SFQ – factor analysis – 4 items
Mascola et al. (2010)	USA	3–11	13–22	Single item
Jin et al. (2009)	China	1–6	39.7	Study-specific questionnaire
Jacobi et al. (2008) [14]	Germany	11.7–12.7	19 (girls) 18 (boys)	Single item
Dubois et al. (2007)	Canada	Preschoolers	14–17	Three items
Wright et al. (2007)	UK	1.5	8.3	Single item
Carruth et al. (2004) [9]	USA	24 months	50	Single item
Jacobi et al. (2003)	USA	3–4	21	SFQ – 4 items
Cerro et al. (2002)	New Zealand	31 months	20	Study-specific questionnaire
Reau et al. (1996)	USA	13–27	36	Single item
Rydell et al. (1995)	Sweden	6.1–11.0	30	Three items

CEBL, Child Behaviour Checklist; CEBQ, Children's Eating Behaviour Questionnaire; CFQ, Child Feeding Questionnaire; LBC, Lifestyle Behaviour Checklist; SFQ, Stanford Feeding Questionnaire.

psychological factors or physical factors, such as swallowing difficulties. The assessment and management of these interacting factors is shown in Figure 1 [8].

The global prevalence of picky eating is estimated to vary greatly, from 5.6% in 4-year-olds in the Netherlands to 50% in 2-year-olds in the USA [9, 10]. A study conducted on Chinese children aged between 7 and 12 years reported a high prevalence rate of 59%. However, it should be noted that the category was overrepresented due to the inclusion of children who were described as "somewhat picky" and those who were "always picky" [11]. The wide range of prevalence in picky eating can be attributed to the variations in its definition and the differences in the methods of assessment used.

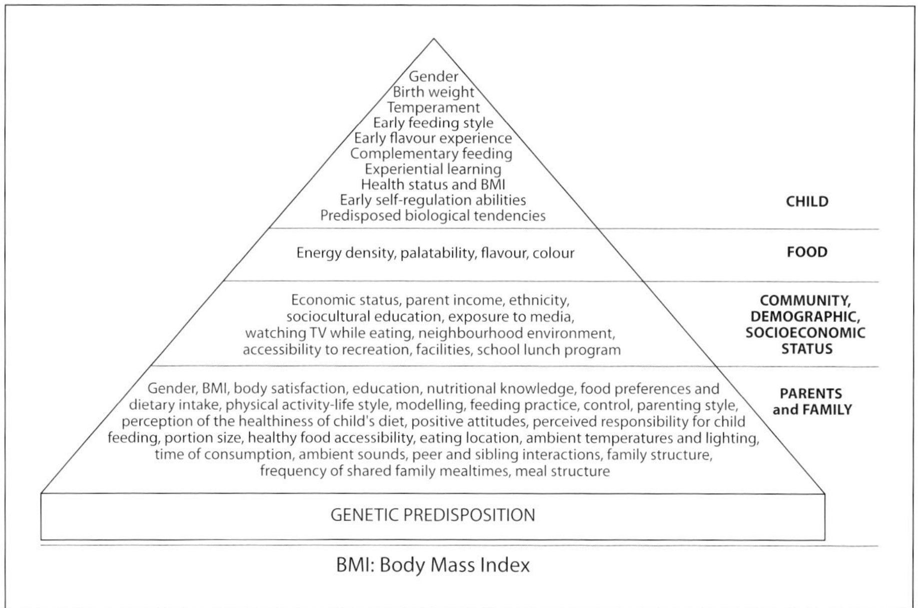

Fig. 1. Decision tree to assess and manage feeding difficulties in children. GI, gastrointestinal; OT, occupational therapist; SLP, speech and language pathologist.

According to their caregivers or physicians, the percentage of children with feeding or eating problems is relatively high worldwide. The prevalence of picky eating behaviors and feeding difficulties varies widely between studies, ranging from 6% to 50% [6, 7]. For example, a survey conducted among households with infants and toddlers aged between four and 24 months showed that the percentage of children identified as picky eaters by their caregivers increased from 19% to 50% as the children's age increased from four to 24 months. Picky eaters were found in all age ranges, both sexes, all ethnicities, and all ranges of household incomes. The survey revealed that older children were more likely to be selective with food choices [9].

The impact of selective eating during childhood is primarily reflected in its effect on overall dietary intake. Picky eating may reduce food intake, resulting in an imbalanced nutrient intake and poor dietary diversity [12], which in turn can lead to adverse health and developmental outcomes.

The amount of research exploring the effects of picky eating on dietary diversity and variety is relatively low. However, studies have demonstrated that at 24–36 months of age, picky eaters consume fewer different food items and have less variety in their food choices, compared to less picky eaters [13]. There is a correlation between selective eating habits and various negative behavioral consequences that impact externalizing and internalizing behaviors [14].

Several studies have shown that picky eating is associated with a greater risk of being underweight and having poor growth. This is likely to be driven by lower energy intake, in combination with low intakes of micronutrients such as zinc and iron, which are critical for optimal growth [15].

Poor Access to a Balanced Diet

Picky eating can lead to malnutrition in cases where there is a significantly low nutrient intake. However, access to food is also a significant predictor of malnutrition and MNDs.

In 2022, there were an estimated 45 million children under 5 suffering from wasting resulting from poor nutrient intake [16]. Malnutrition in infants and young children can be associated with a higher risk of infectious diseases, such as respiratory tract infections.

The WHO also highlights being overweight as a form of malnutrition as this is often associated with high intake of nutrient-poor ultra-processed foods [16]. This may increase the risk of MNDs due to an imbalanced diet intake.

Dietary Solutions

Dietary solutions can be targeted at an individual level, for example supporting parents of children with picky eating, or by providing stand-alone supplementation to be used alongside existing food intake in those at risk of malnutrition.

Interventions can also be at a population level, such as fortification of frequently consumed products to reduce MNDs on a wider scale. This may improve MNDs related to malnutrition by optimizing the nutritional composition of the foods that are available to these population groups.

Individual-Level Solutions

Children who have severe feeding difficulties are at a higher risk of experiencing nutritional deficiencies, poor growth, cognitive impairment, emotional dysfunction, and even death [5]. Early identification of feeding issues and timely intervention can improve outcomes for children [5].

Research findings suggest that parents play a crucial role in improving their children's dietary habits from an early age. To achieve this, parents should focus on incorporating more nutrient-rich and fiber-rich foods, mainly fruits and vegetables, into their children's diets for long-term benefits [12]. This requires strategies that provide education for parents alongside support from healthcare professionals.

Successfully feeding young children requires a good understanding of nutrition by the caregiver or parent. This ensures that the foods offered, the feeding practices, and the calorie amounts provided are appropriate. Presently, intervention studies that identify ways to improve children's eating behaviors are limited. The strategies that exist are age-specific and not based on evidence.

However, valuable insights into parental practices can be obtained from cross-sectional and observational studies, summarized in Table 2. Children's eating behavior and choices are influenced mainly by their parents' dietary habits and feeding techniques. Parents should introduce their children to nutritious food options and balanced diets and set a good example by being positive role models [17].

UNICEF recommends feeding children with feeding difficulties healthy foods when hungry. Children should be allowed to feed themselves to feel in control of what they eat. Rewarding or punishing with food should be avoided. Frequent and smaller meals throughout the day are recommended. Milk and water are better than sugary drinks. Distractions should be avoided during mealtimes, and family eating routines can make mealtime fun [18].

Pediatricians can benefit from understanding the mechanisms that underlie food habits in children. This knowledge can aid in promoting healthy eating practices among children. Therefore, the study of children's behavior can serve as a foundation for developing targeted and effective nutrition education programs. It also suggests the need for further research to explore the interactions between various factors that influence children's eating behaviors [17] (shown in Fig. 2) [19].

Individually tailored dietary supplements can also effectively address micronutrient inadequacies and deficiencies. In Asia, for example, supplementing children under two with vitamin A is a well-established strategy to prevent irreversible blindness that may result from deficiency during early childhood [20]. However, low compliance seems to be a common challenge worldwide.

Data suggest that only 8.8% of infants in India received the appropriate vitamin D supplementation in terms of dose, frequency, and duration [21]. The percentage of infants in the United States who were given oral vitamin D supplements was also low, regardless of whether they were consuming breast milk or formula. The rate ranged from 1% to 13% and varied depending on the infants' age, which ranged from 1 to 10.5 months [22]. In France, only 41.5%–66.6% of the vitamin D prescriptions for children between 0 and 5 years old complied with the recommendations [23]. This would leave a question mark about the effectiveness of widely used strategies to prevent MNDs.

Table 2. Effective strategies and practices to improve children's eating behavior

Strategy	Practices
Covert control	• Buy only healthy foods for home • Avoid unhealthy and fast-food stores
Avoid the use of food rewards	• Food maintains the behaviour on which its delivery and acquisition is dependent
Promoting self-regulation	• Sense of fullness recognition • Serve moderate portions • Assist with organizing the feeding environment
Authoritative parenting style	• Encourage the child to try new foods • Parents are the example • Parents demonstrate the importance of healthy food while also enjoying it • Do not model disliking of foods in front of the child • Parents must control their children's consumption of palatable snack foods in an obesogenic environment • Early responsive parenting intervention
Parent's focused intervention	• Interventions based on education that are tailored for parents and caregivers • Feeding-related advice • Empowering parents • Social support
Family meals	• Expose the child to a variety of foods • Offer the child food repeatedly • Allow the child to have input into food choices • High frequency of shared family meals • Daily shared breakfast • Socialization during mealtime • Turn off the TV at meals
Family environment	• Exposure to healthy tastes and flavors during early life may encourage healthy eating habits • Give the parental role in food shopping and preparation • Healthy food availability • Get Adequate sleep • Reduce screen time

Home fortification strategies are an innovation aimed at improving the diet quality of the nutritionally vulnerable groups, such as young children [24]. There are several methods to increase the overall nutritional value of everyday meals, compared to supplementation with one specific nutrient as outlined above.

One of these methods is the food-first approach, which involves using everyday foods and drinks for meals. Another method is home food fortification, the easiest and most effective way to add oral nutritional supplements to regular meals during preparation. This method helps increase the nutritional value of everyday meals and can address potential challenges such as palatability, compliance, and cost. The oral nutritional supplements contain protein, carbohydrates, fats, vitamins, and minerals, making them a simple and easy way to fortify meals. They are typically used by individuals who struggle to meet their nutrition and hydration needs through an oral diet alone. These individuals are usually at nutritional risk and have been identified using a validated malnutrition screening tool [25].

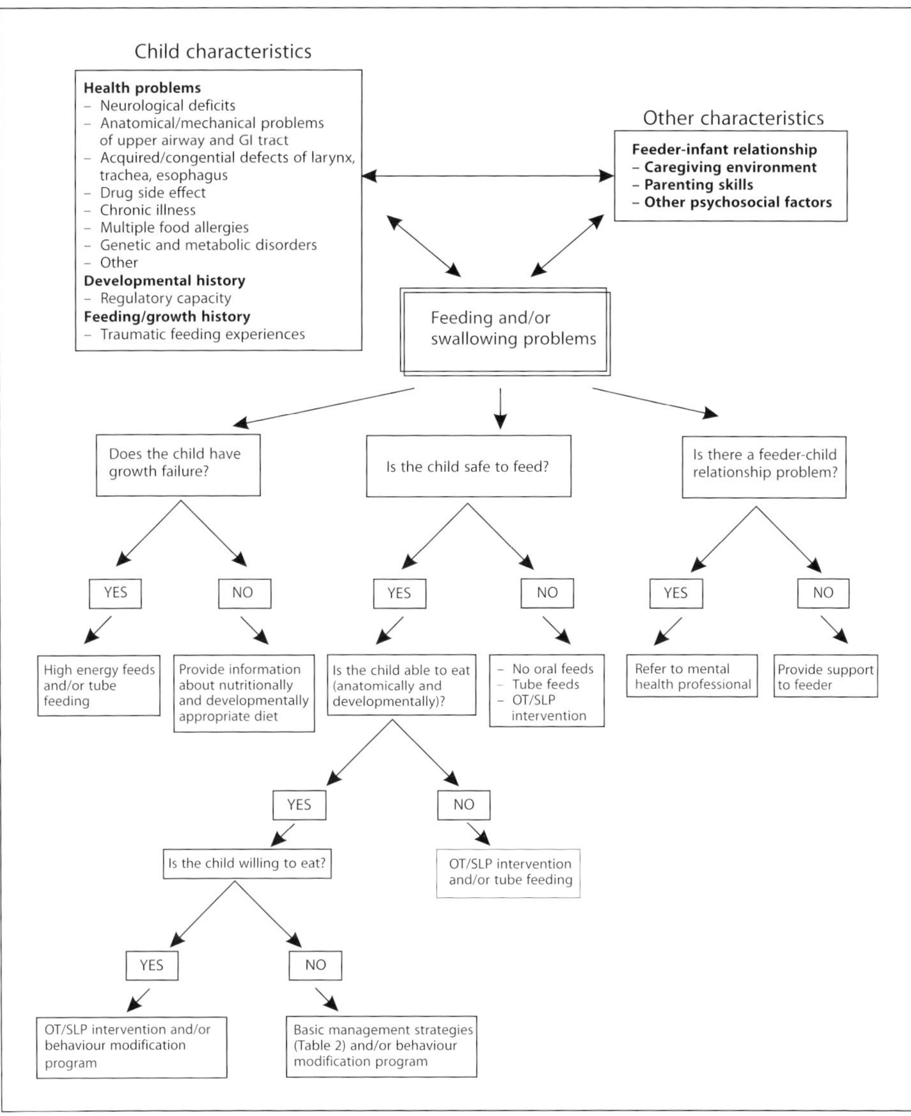

Fig. 2. Factors influencing children's eating behavior.

Population-Level Solutions

MNDs related to malnutrition may also be preventable through food fortification at a population level. Several countries have been fortifying foods since the 1920s, resulting in the eradication of nutrition-related diseases.

Specialized nutritious foods have been developed to meet the higher nutrient needs of specific target groups.

Food fortification adds vitamins and minerals to food during processing to increase its nutritional value. It is an effective and safe strategy to improve diets and prevent and control micronutrient deficiencies. In 2008 and 2012, the Copenhagen Consensus rated food fortification as one of the most cost-effective development priorities [26].

Several factors, such as the high occurrence of specific MNDs, the populations that are most impacted, dietary composition, available infrastructure, food processing, and production systems, as well as national regulation and governmental leadership, determine the most appropriate and effective type of fortification for a given country [27]. Unlike in Western countries, commercial or Industrial Food fortification in low-income countries, the Middle East for example, is sporadic and ineffective; therefore, a review of alternative interventions is required, as well as collaborative changes at policy levels [28].

The World Food Programme committed to increasing the proportion of fortified wheat flour, maize meal, and rice distributed through its programs from 60% in 2020 to 80% in 2025. The World Food Programme will work with at least 40 countries to ensure national systems can bring fortified foods within reach of the most vulnerable families [29].

Point-of-use fortification refers to adding vitamins and minerals to food that is already cooked and ready to be consumed. This method was previously known as "home fortification," but the WHO changed the term to "point-of-use" in 2012 to reflect the various settings where this intervention can occur, such as in schools and refugee camps. In 2016, the WHO recommended using micronutrient powders to fortify complementary foods at the point of use as a crucial step in improving the intake of micronutrients, particularly iron, and reducing anemia in children aged 6 to 24 months [30].

Conclusion

Inadequate dietary intake and malnutrition can be caused by factors including eating behaviors or poor access to food. Food fortification has the potential to address malnutrition globally in a cost-effective way. Studies have shown that fortifying foods at an individual or population level can yield positive results, particularly in controlling and preventing micronutrient deficiencies among vulnerable populations, such as children.

Conflict of Interest Statement

The author has no conflicts of interest to declare.

Funding Sources

The author received lecture honoraria and travel reimbursement from Nestlé Nutrition Institute.

References

1 WHO. Micronutrients. Available from: https://www.who.int/health-topics/micronutrients#tab=tab_1 (June 17, 2024).
2 WHO, GHS U. The state of the world's children 2009: maternal and newborn health. Children. 2009:1–168.
3 Kotecha PV Micronutrient malnutrition in India: let us say "no" to it now. Indian J Community Med 2008; 33:9–10. https://dx.doi.org/10.4103/0970-0218.39235
4 McCormick V, Markowitz G. Picky eater or feeding disorder? Strategies for determining the difference. Adv NPs PAs. 2013;4:18–23.
5 Dovey TM, Staples PA, Gibson EL, Halford JCG. Food neophobia and 'picky/fussy' eating in children: a review. Appetite. 2008;50:181–93. https://dx.doi.org/10.1016/j.appet.2007.09.009
6 Goh DYT, Jacob A. Perception of picky eating among children in Singapore and its impact on caregivers: a questionnaire survey. Asia Pac Fam Med. 2012;11:5. https://doi.org/10.1186/1447-056X-11-5
7 Taylor CM, Wernimont SM, Northstone K, Emmett PM. Picky/fussy eating in children: review of definitions, assessment, prevalence and dietary intakes. Appetite [Internet]. 2015; 95:349–59. https://dx.doi.org/10.1016/j.appet.2015.07.026
8 Arts-Rodas D, Benoit D. Feeding problems in infancy and early childhood: identification and management. Paediatr Child Health. 1998;3:21–7. https://dx.doi.org/10.1093/pch/3.1.21
9 Carruth BR, Ziegler PJ, Gordon A, Barr SI. Prevalence of picky eaters among infants and toddlers 'and their caregivers' decisions about offering a new food. J Am Diet Assoc. 2004;104:s57–64. https://dx.doi.org/10.1016/j.jada.2003.10.024
10 Tharner A, Jansen PW, Kiefte-de Jong JC, Moll HA, van der Ende J, Jaddoe VWV, et al. Toward an operative diagnosis of fussy/picky eating: a latent profile approach in a population-based cohort. Int J Behav Nutr Phys Act [Internet]. 2014;11:14. https://doi.org/10.1186/1479-5868-11-14
11 Xue Y, Lee E, Ning K, Zheng Y, Ma D, Gao H, et al. Prevalence of picky eating behaviour in Chinese school-age children and associations with anthropometric parameters and intelligence quotient. A cross-sectional study. Appetite [Internet]. 2015;91:248–55. https://dx.doi.org/10.1016/j.appet.2015.04.065
12 Taylor CM, Emmett PM. Picky eating in children: causes and consequences. Proc Nutr Soc. 2019;78:161–9. https://dx.doi.org/10.1017/S0029665118002586
13 Cardona Cano CS, Tiemeier H, Van Hoeken D, Tharner A, Jaddoe VWV, Hofman A, et al Trajectories of picky eating during childhood: a general population study. Int J Eat Disord. 2015; 48:570–9. https://dx.doi.org/10.1002/eat.22384
14 Jacobi C, Schmitz G, Agras WS. Is picky eating an eating disorder? Int J Eat Disord [Internet]. 2008;41:626–34. https://dx.doi.org/10.1002/eat.20545
15 Taylor CM, Northstone K, Wernimont SM, Emmett PM. Macro- and micronutrient intakes in picky eaters: a cause for concern? Am J Clin Nutr. 2016;104:1647–56. https://dx.doi.org/10.3945/ajcn.116.137356
16 United Nations Children's Fund (UNICEF), World Health Organization (WHO), International Bank for Reconstruction and Development/The World Bank. Levels and trends in child malnutrition: UNICEF/WHO/World Bank Group Joint Child Malnutrition estimates: key findings of the 2023 edition. New York: UNICEF and WHO; 2023. CC BY-NC-SA 3.0 IGO.
17 Scaglioni S, De Cosmi V, Ciappolino V, Parazzini F, Brambilla P, Agostoni C. Factors influencing children's eating behaviours. Nutrients. 2018;10. https://dx.doi.org/10.3390/nu10060706
18 Care and feeding for children with feeding difficulties. IYCF Image Bank [Internet]. [cited 2024 Apr 1]. Available from: https://iycfimagebank.org/cards/1027/7

19 De Cosmi V, Scaglioni S, Agostoni C. Early taste experiences and later food choices. Nutrients. 2017;9(2):107. https://doi.org/10.3390/nu9020107
20 Trentmann C. Supplementation, food fortification and dietary diversification. BMZ; 2012. p. 1–10.
21 Meena P, Saran AN, Shah D, Gupta P. Compliance to prescription of routine vitamin D supplementation in infants. Indian Pediatr. 2020;57:1067–9. https://dx.doi.org/10.1007/s13312-020-2037-x
22 Perrine CG, Sharma AJ, Jefferds MED, Serdula MK, Scanlon KS. Adherence to vitamin D recommendations among US infants. Pediatrics. 2010;125:627–32. https://dx.doi.org/10.1542/peds.2009-2571
23 Mallet E, Gaudelus J, Reinert P, Stagnara J, Bénichou J, Castanet M, et al [Prophylactic prescription of vitamin D in France: national multicenter epidemiological study of 3240 children under 6 years of age]. Arch Pediatr. 2012;19: 1293–302. https://dx.doi.org/10.1016/j.arcped.2012.09.011
24 De-Regil LM, Suchdev PS, Vist GE, Walleser S, Peña-Rosas JP. Home fortification of foods with multiple micronutrient powders for health and nutrition in children under two years of age. Cochrane Database Syst Rev. 2011;CD008959. https://dx.doi.org/10.1002/14651858.CD008959.pub2
25 The importance of a food first approach. Nualtra [Internet]. [cited 2024 Apr 1]. Available from: https://nualtra.com/resources/news/the-importance-of-a-food-first-approach
26 Hoddinott J, Rosegrant M, Torero M. HUNGER AND MALNUTRITION Investments to reduce hunger and undernutrition; 2012.
27 Olson R, Gavin-Smith B, Ferraboschi C, Kraemer K. Food fortification: the advantages, disadvantages and lessons from sight and life programs. Nutrients. 2021;13(4). https://dx.doi.org/10.3390/nu13041118
28 Hwalla N, Al Dhaheri AS, Radwan H, Alfawaz HA, Fouda MA, Al-Daghri NM, et al. The prevalence of micronutrient deficiencies and inadequacies in the Middle East and approaches to interventions. Nutrients. 2017;9. https://dx.doi.org/10.3390/nu9030229
29 Food fortification. World Food Programme [Internet]. [cited 2024 Apr 1]. Available from: https://www.wfp.org/food-fortification
30 World Health Organization. WHO guideline: use of multiple micronutrient powders for point-of-use fortification of foods consumed by infants and young children aged 6–23 Months and children aged 2–12 years. World Heal Organ [Internet]. 2016 [cited 2024 Apr 1];Licence: CC BY-NC-SA 3.0 IGO. Available from: https://www.ncbi.nlm.nih.gov/books/NBK409165/

Eslam Tawfik ElBaroudy
Department of Pediatrics, Faculty of Medicine
Suez University
Suez, Egypt
Elbaroudy75@yahoo.com

Published online: November 15, 2024

Szajewska H, Neu J, Shamir R, Wong G, Prentice AM (eds): Shaping the Future with Nutrition. Nestle Nutr Inst Workshop Ser. Basel, Karger, 2024, vol 100, pp 111–124 (DOI: 10.1159/000540141)

Micronutrient Hunger or Hidden Hunger Among Infants and Young Children on Healthy Diets

George Jacob Elizabeth[a] Gibby Koshy[b]

[a]Department of Pediatrics, Ananthapuri Hospitals & Research Institute, Thiruvananthapuram, India; [b]Parkview Family Health Care Centre, Kundara, India

Abstract

"Hidden Hunger" refers to micronutrient deficiencies that are not necessarily reflected in anthropometric measurements and thus remain hidden. It affects 2 billion people globally, and occurs among infants and young children on a "healthy diet," as perceived by family members. Hidden hunger is recognizable with a high index of suspicion and hence the term "micronutrient hunger" has been proposed. Its effects are significant and include physical and mental impairment, poor health, low productivity, morbidity, and mortality. Data reported in the Global Hunger Index and Global Hidden Hunger Index are eye-openers in this context. Maternal deficiencies, changing breastfeeding trends, suboptimum infant and young child feeding practices, and universal availability and popularization of junk food result in emerging and re-emerging nutritional disorders that need to be addressed urgently. Strategies for addressing micronutrient malnutrition include supplementation, fortification, and dietary diversification. These interventions have benefits but are limited by context and resources. In the Indian context, universal salt iodization is successful; however, iron and folic acid supplementation for several decades has not produced the desired results. A multisectoral approach advocated at national and international levels with cross-disciplinary support is recommended. An overview of these issues along with practical solutions are highlighted in this manuscript.

Introduction

The term "hidden hunger" refers to the deficiency of micronutrients such as essential minerals and vitamins, which are not visible at first sight [1]. Deficiencies are often undetected, especially in infants and young children, but can be recognized if a high suspicion index exists. A majority of the deficiencies have important public health consequences. Therefore, the term "micronutrient hunger" has been proposed instead of "hidden hunger." Hidden hunger affects more than 2 billion people, which accounts for one-third of the population worldwide [2]. Its effects can be significant, leading to impaired physical growth, poor cognitive function, learning disabilities, chronic diseases, low productivity, and even death.

Global Hunger Index and Global Hidden Hunger Index

The Global Hunger Index (GHI) is a tool created to track and measure hunger worldwide by nation and region. India is ranked 107th, with a reported GHI prevalence of 29%, a mere 10% decrease from 39% in 2000 [3]. The target of "Zero Hunger by 2030" is still far off without swift, long-lasting, and significant improvements.

Each nation's GHI score is computed based on the four indicators that collectively reflect the multifaceted character of hunger. GHI scores are obtained as a result of the computation, with 0 being the best score (no hunger) and 100 representing the worst. The four component indicators listed below are combined to calculate GHI [3]:

- Undernourishment: the proportion of the population consuming insufficient amounts of calories.
- Child stunting: the proportion of children under 5 years who have low height for their age, a sign of chronic undernutrition.
- Child wasting: the proportion of young children under 5 years who are underweight for their height, a sign of acute undernutrition.
- Child mortality: the percentage of children who died before turning 5 years old, partly due to the lethal combination of poor diet and unhygienic surroundings.

Deficiencies of four micronutrients – iron, iodine, zinc, and vitamin A – pose the greatest threat to global public health because of their rising prevalence and the ensuing negative effects on development and health.

The Global Hidden Hunger Index (GHHI) 2022 focuses on micronutrients as a part of the dramatic hunger situation worldwide. It is measured among preschool-age children as the average of three deficiency prevalence estimates: (i) stunting due to zinc deficiency, (ii) anemia due to iron deficiency, and (iii) vitamin A deficiency.

Zinc serves as a surrogate for stunting, iron for physical capability and cognition, and vitamin A for immunity. In the Hidden Hunger Index in preschool children score, these three components are equally weighted: ([stunting (%) + anemia (%) + low serum retinol (%)]/3) [4].

Micronutrient deficits, or hidden hunger, are often intergenerational. Due to their prevalence among adolescents, particularly girls, it is often passed down to the next generation. Hidden hunger is often associated with lowered or compromised immunity and growth, which may eventually lead to degenerative and chronic illnesses. According to the 2019 report “Adolescents, Diets and Nutrition: Growing Well in a Changing World” by UNICEF over 80% of the adolescent population in India demonstrated multiple micronutrient deficiencies [5]. Increasing incomes and changes in dietary patterns among adolescents with greater consumption of junk foods, fried foods, and sugar-sweetened beverages and less consumption of green leafy vegetables and fruits are contributing to this nutritional disaster.

Infant and Young Child Feeding Practices

Optimum complementary foods; adequate supplementary feeding techniques, such as meal frequency and nutritional diversity; and enough nutrition services are the factors that determine young children’s diets during the complementary feeding period. A child’s right to have a wholesome, secure, reasonably priced, and sustainable diet is predicted by the determinants and drivers of their nutrition in their early years. These diets, in turn, contribute to protecting, promoting, and supporting growth, development, and survival [6]. It is important to emphasize that a nutritious diet in a child starts with exclusive breastfeeding as it serves as the cornerstone for long-term health benefits, including reducing the risk of obesity or the later onset of noncommunicable diseases. The complementary feeding period is also critical as it is challenging to cater to an infant’s high nutritional needs and quick physiological changes during this time [6].

Children between the ages of 6 and 23 months have greater nutritional needs per kilogram of body weight for growth and development. To ensure adequate nutrition, it’s crucial to offer children a diverse range of foods regularly. However, data indicate that most toddlers between the ages of 6 and 23 months are not fed per global norms as shown in Figure 1a–c [7]. In addition, many children neither get the proper nutrition at the right age nor have enough variety

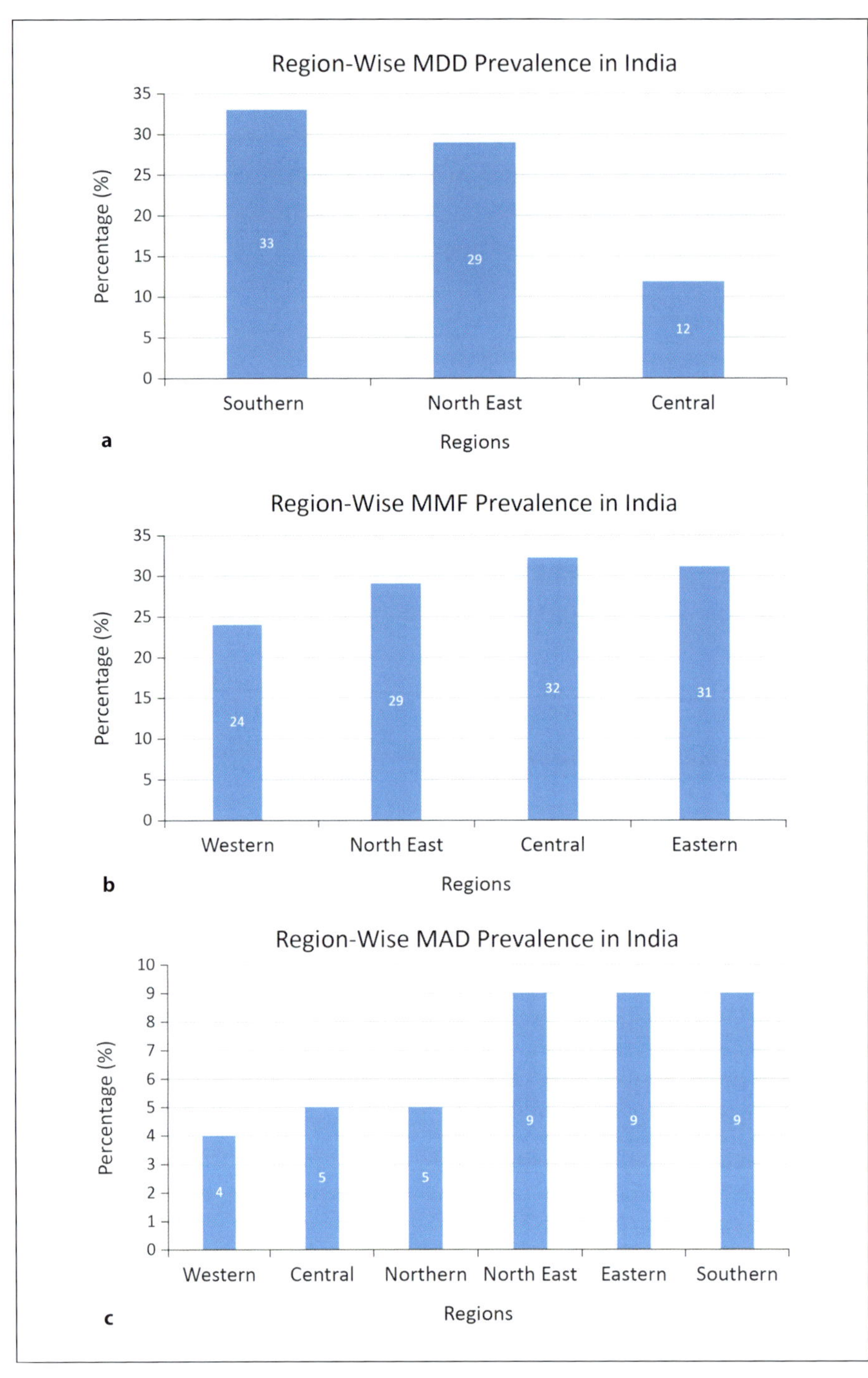

Fig. 1. a MDD prevalence in India. **b** MMF prevalence in India. **c** MAD prevalence in India [7]. MAD, minimum acceptable diet; MDD, minimum dietary diversity; MMF, minimum meal frequency.

in their diets to help them reach their maximum potential in terms of growth and development. When a child lacks a necessary vitamin, they either develop faster and use up more body stores, which eventually causes a loss in bodily functions (type I functional nutrients), or they grow slower and actively conserve the nutrient to keep the concentration in the tissues (type II functional nutrients) [8]. The list of type I and type II nutrients is shown in Table 1 [8].

Inadequate feeding practices can result in various deficiencies in children, even when energy intake remains adequate due to consuming energy-dense but nutrient-poor foods [2]. Some reasons for hidden hunger are reliance on low-cost, monotonous staples, limited choices, lack of dietary diversity of foods, impaired absorption or use of nutrients, and the presence of antinutrients, which limit the bioavailability of nutrients that are crucial for growth and development [9].

Healthy Diets and Micronutrient Deficiencies

Various deficiencies have been reported among infants and young children while on a so-called "healthy diet." Several emerging and re-emerging nutritional disorders such as nutritional cardiomyopathy and cardiac failure due to deficiencies in iron, thiamine, selenium, and vitamin D are not uncommon. Changes in myocardial energy generation, calcium balance, or oxidative defenses are linked to long-term deficiencies in thiamine, carnitine, selenium, niacin, taurine, and coenzyme Q10 in the cardiac tissues [10]. Recently, a condition known as thiamine-responsive acute pulmonary hypertension of early infancy has been recognized in many parts of India among exclusively breastfed infants, who eminently respond to thiamine [11]. Exclusive breastfeeding by thiamine-deficient but otherwise asymptomatic mothers is one of the key risk

Table 1. Type I and Type II nutrients [8]

Type I nutrients	Type II nutrients
Iron	Nitrogen
Iodine	Essential amino acids
Copper	Potassium
Calcium	Magnesium
Selenium	Phosphorus
Thiamine	Sulfur
Riboflavin	Zinc
Pyridoxine	Sodium
Niacin	Chloride
Folate	
Cobalamin	
Vitamins A, D, E, and K	

factors for thiamine-responsive acute pulmonary hypertension in early infancy. Mothers who consume only polished wheat products without any bran of the cereals may have severe thiamine deficiency. The clinical features include acute respiratory distress, cardiomegaly, gross right ventricle dilatation, pulmonary arterial hypertension, and metabolic acidosis and shock [11].

Infantile tremor syndrome and megaloblastic anemia with hyperpigmentation of periungual and knuckle regions and delayed developmental milestones due to vitamin B_{12} deficiency have been identified among exclusively breastfed infants [12]. Previous studies have shown a causal relationship between infantile tremor syndrome and vitamin B_{12} insufficiency among mothers who were B_{12} deficient, especially those who followed a strict vegan diet [12]. In certain regions of India and within specific communities, strict adherence to vegetarian or vegan diets is widespread. Infants born to vegan mothers may lack sufficient vitamin B_{12} stores, making them vulnerable to developing infantile B_{12} deficiency. This deficiency can lead to developmental delays, neuro-regression, infantile tremors, and megaloblastic anemia. However, clinical symptoms may take years to appear, but they often improve with vitamin B_{12} therapy.

The association between folic acid deficiency and fetal neural tube defects is well documented [13]. Folate deficiency is widespread and leads to megaloblastic anemia and dimorphic anemia, along with associated iron deficiency. Maternal folate deficiency increases the risk of neural tube defect (NTD) in the offspring in the general population. As a majority of women are not aware of their pregnancies until 21–28 days following conception, which is when these abnormalities arise, folate supplementation is necessary as a preconception intervention. Data from 1,242 children with NTDs were compared with data from a control group of 6,660 infants with deformities unrelated to vitamin supplementation. The adjusted odds ratios of NTDs related to exposure to carbamazepine during the first or second month after the last menstrual period, compared with no use in either month were 6.9 (95% confidence interval: 1.9, 25.7) for carbamazepine (6 exposed cases). The discovery that folic acid had no discernible protective effect in mothers taking antiepileptic medications was equally startling. These findings imply that antiepileptic drugs disrupt folate metabolism at different levels. Folic acid supplementation for a long period or at high levels during the preconception period might lower the likelihood of birth abnormalities [14]. It is also crucial to ensure vitamin B_{12} sufficiency while supplementing folic acid in pregnant women. Vitamin B_{12} helps in retrieving the active form tetrahydrofolate from an inactive metabolite, N (5)-methyl-tetrahydrofolate. This phenomenon known as the "folate trap," leads to aggravation of vitamin B_{12} deficiency in already deficient individuals [15]. Zinc deficiency is quite widespread among infants and young children and is often suspected in those with persistent diarrhea and acrodermatitis, even though the genetic defect resulting from this condition is rare [16]. Excess zinc, however, can have counter effects on the "twin minerals" iron and copper.

Iron deficiency is widespread across all age groups, resulting in microcytic hypochromic anemia with reduced physical stamina and cognition and a higher incidence of febrile convulsions, breath-holding spells, and restless leg syndrome [17, 18]. Iron excess can lead to hemochromatosis through the generation of free radicals. The occurrence of Pica disorders such as geophagia (mud), amylophagia (raw rice), and pagophagia (ice) in children suggests iron deficiency anemia. Iron deficiency is rampant, and sufficiency is difficult to achieve due to the low bioavailability of non-heme iron and the presence of antinutrients such as phytates, polyphenols, caffeine, and tannin in the diet. Excess consumption of milk, which is considered "healthy" can result in iron deficiency due to cow's milk protein enteropathy [19]. Vitamin C deficiency is a common deficiency encountered in children. Total avoidance of fresh fruits due to fear of pesticides has recently been associated with vitamin C deficiency and scurvy [20].

Lack of sun exposure and to a much lesser extent, lack of intake of fatty food, are the causes for the re-emergence of vitamin D deficiency and rickets [21]. These conditions are rampant and are considered emerging lifestyle-related diseases, even in countries such as India where sunlight is abundant. Lack of sun exposure around noon time, environmental pollution, lifestyle changes, way of dressing and use of sunscreens, and inadequate dietary intake are some of the contributing factors. As vitamin D is a fat-soluble vitamin, overzealous supplementation can result in hypervitaminosis D. Other micronutrient deficiencies are fluorosis, a re-emerging disease due to excess fluoride in drinking water [22]; vitamin A deficiency; and iodine deficiency. In summary, maternal deficiencies, changing breastfeeding trends, suboptimum Infant and Young Child Feeding practices, and universal availability and popularization of junk food result in emerging and re-emerging nutritional disorders, which need to be addressed urgently.

Impact of Micronutrient Malnutrition

Hidden hunger in developing countries is associated with negative effects on health and survival [23]. Micronutrient deficiencies affect people directly and society indirectly. There are widespread micronutrient deficiencies in the world, with pregnant women and their unborn children being most at risk [24]. Micronutritional deficits rarely occur alone, and deficits of different micronutrients frequently coexist in an individual. The long-term effects of micronutrient deficiencies are detrimental to national economic development and human

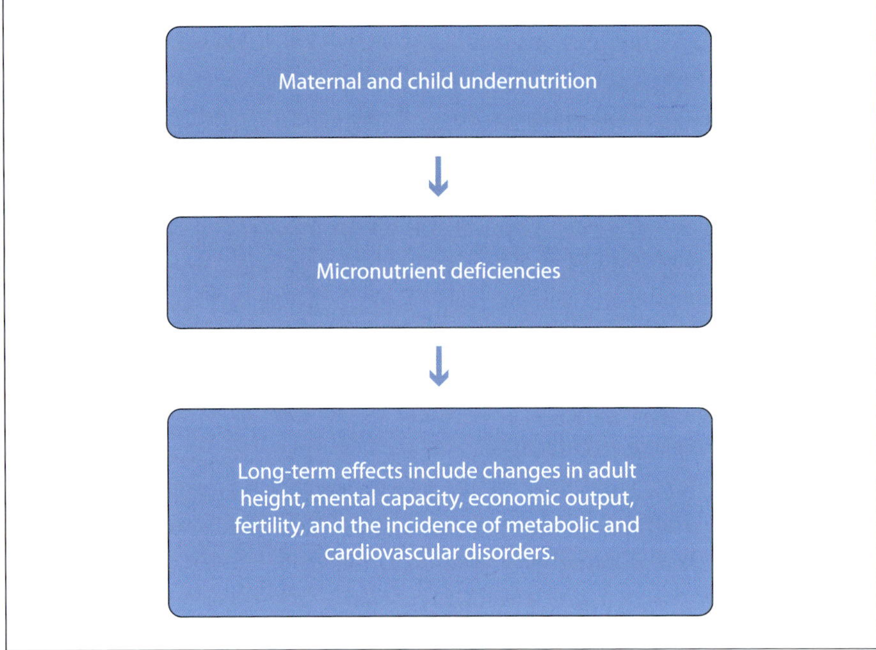

Fig. 2. Long-lasting impact of micronutrient deficiencies [24].

capital in addition to being evident at the individual level [24]. The intergenerational effects of micronutrient deficiencies, which we are only now beginning to comprehend, and the cycle of micronutrient deficiencies that last throughout generations must be of utmost concern [24].

Micronutrient deficiencies can have long-lasting implications as depicted in Figure 2.

Strategies to Tackle Micronutrient Malnutrition

The goal of increasing food production to satisfy the demands of the world's expanding population has centered on efficiency and yield maximization. The output of energy has increased, while the micronutrient content of diets has decreased. As a result, several strategies have been used to raise micronutrient intake:

- Supplementation
- Fortification
- Biofortification
- Diversification of diet

While there are benefits to each intervention, their effectiveness is contingent upon the specific environment and resources at hand. A multisectoral approach at the national and international levels is required to successfully address the problem of improving the diets of young children during the supplemental feeding phase.

Micronutrient Supplementation

The fastest improvement in the micronutrient status of individuals or targeted populations typically results from supplementation, which is the administration of high quantities of micronutrients in a highly absorbable form [25]. Although supplementation programs are initially used as short-term measure to tackle hidden hunger, these are then usually replaced by long-term sustainable measures like dietary modification and food fortification usually by increasing dietary diversity. India is running universal and targeted supplementation with micronutrients such as iron; folic acid; iodine; zinc; and vitamins A, D, K, and B_{12}. The "United Nations International Multiple Micronutrient Antenatal Preparation" is a novel multiple micronutrient supplementation strategy that includes 15 nutrients [26], which is recommended by the United Nations for prenatal mothers as shown in Table 2. However, it is yet to be implemented globally.

Commercial Food Fortification

Commercial food fortification, which refers to the addition of micronutrients to processed foods, is a broad, integrated approach to prevent hidden hunger. It is an important tool to support and reinforce existing nutrition programs and

Table 2. Multiple micronutrient supplement formulation [26]

Component	Chemical entity	Amount
Vitamin A	Retinyl acetate	800 μg RAE
Vitamin C	Ascorbic acid	70 mg
Vitamin D	Cholecalciferol	5 μg (200 IU)
Vitamin E	Alpha tocopheryl succinate	10 mg α-TE
Vitamin B_1	Thiamine mononitrate	1.4 mg
Vitamin B_2	Riboflavin	1.4 mg
Vitamin B_3	Niacinamide	18 mg NE
Vitamin B_6	Pyridoxine HCl	1.9 mg
Folic acid	Folic acid	680 μg DFE (400 μg)
Vitamin B_{12}	Cyanocobalamin	2.6 μg
Iron	Ferrous fumarate	30 mg
Iodine	Potassium iodide	150 μg
Zinc	Zinc oxide	15 mg
Selenium	Sodium selenite	65 μg
Copper	Cupric oxide	2 mg

could be helpful for the prevention of specific nutritional deficiencies. It has been successful as a cost-effective public health strategy for promoting overall well-being. Iodization of salt, and the addition of B-complex vitamins, zinc, and iron to wheat flour and vitamin A to sugar and cooking oil are other good examples of food fortification. Iron and iodine double-fortified salt is also under trial in India. Fortified rice kernel, including iron folic acid and vitamin B_{12}, added to rice in a ratio of 1:100 is being supplied in supplementary feeding programs in India.

Biofortification

Biofortification, an emerging intervention, expected to grow significantly, enhances nutritional content in crops using transgenic methods [27]. Biofortified foods provide a safe and steady source of essential micronutrients, which is not available from other interventions. Biofortified crops are nutritious and drought-resilient. Examples of biofortified crops include iron beans, zinc wheat, rice, and vitamin A cassava and maize.

Dietary Diversification

One of the most important and effective methods of preventing nutritional hunger is increasing dietary diversity. Increasing dietary diversity can address micronutrient deficiencies by incorporating a variety of foods from different food groups over time. Dietary diversity is associated with better child nutritional outcomes [28], even when controlling for socioeconomic factors. High prevalence of poor dietary diversity may be linked to meal-skipping and snacking habits, particularly among adolescents [5, 29].

In most instances, parents and caretakers consider the diet of infants and young children as "healthy," as they often lack information on the 17 key Infant and Young Child Feeding indicators, particularly minimum dietary diversity, minimum meal frequency, and minimum acceptable diet [30]. It is a good strategy to ensure that minimum dietary diversity starts from complementary feeding and it should be universalized and popularized. The eight food groups for 6- to 23-month-old children as per the World Health Organization are presented in Table 3 [31].

At least 5 out of 8 food groups should be added in rotation, after 6 months of age, as per the developmental readiness of the baby and locally prevailing cultural practices [21].

Home-Based Newborn Care and Home-Based Young Child Care are platforms for handholding for breastfeeding and complementary feeding practices in the home environment. The "rice-giving ceremony" called "Annaprasan" is being popularized at 6 months of age to promote the introduction of a variety of

Table 3. MDD indicators for 6–23 months old as per the WHO [31]

Age	Food groups
6–23 months	Breast milk
	Grains, roots, tubers, and plantains
	Pulses (beans, peas, lentils), nuts, and seeds
	Dairy products (milk, infant formula, yogurt, cheese)
	Flesh foods (meat, fish, poultry, organ meats)
	Egg
	Vitamin-A–rich fruits and vegetables
	Other fruits and vegetables

foods after the ceremony. Eleven well-baby visits have been planned at the following stages: <7 days, 6, 10, and 14 weeks, and 6, 9, 12, 18, 24, 30, and 36 months for growth, developmental and nutritional surveillance, and counseling. To promote dietary diversity, fortified rice kernels and iodized salt are being used for feeding in all government-sponsored preschools called "Anganwadis" under the Integrated Child Development Services Scheme. In certain model centers, a large basket is provided for mothers and caregivers to contribute various vegetables and fruits, enhancing feeding diversity. Ensuring food security and appropriate supplements is the key to success [32].

The Scaling Up Nutrition (SUN) strategy 2021–2025 (SUN 3.0) is a good model for cross-sectoral collaboration. This strategy brings people and resources together at the national level to improve nutrition, especially among adolescents and prospective mothers. The United Nations Secretary-General introduced the SUN Movement in 2010 along with four SUN Networks: the SUN Donor Network, the SUN Business Network, the SUN Civil Society Network, and the United Nations Nutrition Network. The essential components of this movement to fight hidden hunger are empowering adolescent females by improving their access to education and ensuring social protection, thus giving women from poor backgrounds access to nutritious food and making them immune from price hikes [33].

Conclusion

Micronutrient hunger is a major public health problem. Although most cases of micronutrient hunger remain "hidden," they are recognizable with a high index of suspicion. This affects more than 2 billion people, almost one in three, worldwide. The effects of micronutrient hunger can be significant, leading to physical growth and mental impairment, poor health, low productivity, and even death. Multiple deficiencies can occur in children while on a healthy diet as perceived by the mother.

Promoting optimum breastfeeding and complementary feeding along with behavioral change communication are important to tackle this challenge. Elimination of micronutrient hunger among children and the adolescent population remains a global challenge. Effective interventional strategies that improve the knowledge of nutrition among adolescents and promote healthy food choices are essential as a protective strategy. It is essential to ensure supplementation and a robust food supply rich in micronutrients to combat this. The solutions include implementation of dietary diversification starting from infancy. Even though adequate nutrition can be provided through a variety of cereals, legumes, animal-source foods, fruits, and vegetables, certain populations such as pregnant women, young children, and adolescents need micronutrient supplementation to solve this complex problem. Other workable strategies include food fortification and biofortification, with a multisectoral approach at the national and international levels.

Acknowledgments

We would like to acknowledge BioQuest Solutions Pvt. Ltd., Bangalore, for providing medical writing and editorial support in the preparation of this manuscript.

Conflict of Interest Statement

The authors have no conflicts of interest to declare.

Funding Sources

The author received lecture honoraria and travel reimbursement from Nestlé Nutrition Institute.

Author Contributions

G.J.E. conceived the concept and provided guidance. G.K. carried out a literature search and drafted the manuscript. Both authors have read and approved the final version of the manuscript.

Data Availability Statement

The data used to support the findings of this study are included in the chapter.

References

1 Burchi F, Fanzo J, Frison E. The role of food and nutrition system approaches in tackling hidden hunger. Int J Environ Res Public Health. 2011; 8(2):358–73. https://doi.org/10.3390/ijerph8020358.

2 Lowe NM. The global challenge of hidden hunger: perspectives from the field. Proc Nutr Soc. 2021; 80(3):283–9. https://doi.org/10.1017/S0029665121000902.

3 Global Hunger Index (GHI). Food systems transformation and local governance [cited 2024 Jan 30]. Available from: www.globalhungerindex.org.

4 Muthayya S, Rah JH, Sugimoto JD, Roos FF, Kraemer K, Black RE. The global hidden hunger indices and maps: an advocacy tool for action. PLoS One. 2013;8(6):e67860. https://doi.org/10.1371/journal.pone.0067860.

5 Sethi V, Lahiri A, Bhanot A, Kumar A, Chopra M, Mishra R, et al. Adolescents, diets and nutrition: growing well in a changing world. The CNNS Thematic Reports. 2019;(1):1–4.

6 UNICEF. Improving young children's diets during the complementary feeding period – UNICEF programming guidance. 2020 [cited 2023 Aug 21]. Available from: https://www.unicef.org/media/93981/file/Complementary-Feeding-Guidance-2020.pdf.

7 Dhami MV, Ogbo FA, Osuagwu UL, Agho KE. Prevalence and factors associated with complementary feeding practices among children aged 6-23 months in India: a regional analysis. BMC Publ Health. 2019;19(1):1034. https://doi.org/10.1186/s12889-019-7360-6.

8 Golden MH. Specific deficiencies versus growth failure: type I and type II nutrients. SCN News. 1995;12:10–4.

9 International Food Policy Research Institute (IFPRI). Addressing the challenge of hidden hunger [cited 2023 Aug 10]. Available from: https://www.ifpri.org/sites/default/files/ghi/2014/feature_1818.html.

10 Albakri A. Nutritional deficiency cardiomyopathy: a review and pooled analysis of pathophysiology, diagnosis and clinical management. Res Rev Insights. 2019;3:1–14. https://doi.org/10.15761/rri.1000149.

11 Panigrahy N, Chirla DK, Shetty R, Shaikh FAR, Kumar PP, Madappa R, et al. Thiamine-responsive acute pulmonary hypertension of early infancy (TRAPHEI)-a case series and clinical review. Children (Basel). 2020;7(11):199. https://doi.org/10.3390/children7110199.

12 Gupta R, Mandliya J, Sonker P, Patil V, Agrawal M, Pathak A. Infantile tremor syndrome: role of Vitamin B12 revisited. J Pediatr Neurosci. 2016; 11(4):305–8. https://doi.org/10.4103/1817-1745.199463.

13 Ferrazzi E, Tiso G, Di Martino D. Folic acid versus 5- methyl tetrahydrofolate supplementation in pregnancy. Eur J Obstet Gynecol Reprod Biol. 2020;253:312–9. https://doi.org/10.1016/j.ejogrb.2020.06.012.

14 Green NS. Folic acid supplementation and prevention of birth defects. J Nutr. 2002;132(8 suppl l):2356S–60S. https://doi.org/10.1093/jn/132.8.2356S.

15 Elizabeth KE. Folate: its biological interactions and strategies to achieve sufficiency without causing excess. Am J Public Health. 2021;111(3):347–9. https://doi.org/10.2105/AJPH.2020.306067.

16 Vuralli D, Tumer L, Hasanoglu A. Zinc deficiency in the pediatric age group is common but underevaluated. World J Pediatr. 2017;13(4):360–6. https://doi.org/10.1007/s12519-017-0007-8.

17 Krishnan R, Geetha S, Elizabeth KE, Anisha AN. Iron status among under-five children with first febrile convulsion and subsequent febrile convulsion. Indian J Child Health. 2018;5(6):397–401. https://doi.org/10.32677/ijch.2018.v05.i06.002.

18 Divya K, Dipika MC, Elizabeth KE, Sanjay KM, Relve PV. Signature of iron deficiency anemia on neurodevelopmental outcome among under five children. Glob J Res Anal. 2023;12(2):169–71.

19 Graczykowska K, Kaczmarek J, Wilczyńska D, Łoś-Rycharska E, Krogulska A. The consequence of excessive consumption of cow's milk: protein-losing enteropathy with anasarca in the course of iron deficiency anemia-case reports and a literature review. Nutrients. 2021;13(3):828. https://doi.org/10.3390/nu13030828.

20 Ceglie G, Macchiarulo G, Marchili MR, Marchesi A, Rotondi Aufiero L, Di Camillo C, et al. Scurvy: still a threat in the well-fed first world? Arch Dis Child. 2019;104(4):381–3. https://doi.org/10.1136/archdischild-2018-315496.

21 Pettifor JM. Calcium and vitamin D metabolism in children in developing countries. Ann Nutr Metab. 2014;64(suppl 2):15–22. https://doi.org/10.1159/000365124.

22 Srivastava S, Flora SJS. Fluoride in drinking water and skeletal fluorosis: a review of the global impact. Curr Environ Health Rep. 2020;7(2):140–6. https://doi.org/10.1007/s40572-020-00270-9.

23 Biesalski HK. Hidden hunger in the developed world [cited 2023 Aug 14]. Available from: https://www.nutri-facts.org/content/dam/nutrifacts/media/media-books/RTGN_chapter_03.pdf.

24 Bailey RL, West KP Jr, Black RE. The epidemiology of global micronutrient deficiencies. Ann Nutr Metab. 2015;66(suppl 2):22–33. https://doi.org/10.1159/000371618.

25 Faber M, Berti C, Smuts M. Prevention and control of micronutrient deficiencies in developing countries: current perspectives. Nutr Diet Suppl. 2014;6:41–57. https://doi.org/10.2147/nds.s43523.

26 Multiple Micronutrient Supplement Technical Advisory Group (MMS-TAG), Micronutrient Forum (MNF). Expert consensus on an open-access United Nations International Multiple Micronutrient Antenatal Preparation-multiple micronutrient supplement product specification. Ann N Y Acad Sci. 2020;1470(1):3–13. https://doi.org/10.1111/nyas.14322.

27 Ofori KF, Antoniello S, English MM, Aryee ANA. Improving nutrition through biofortification-a systematic review. Front Nutr. 2022;9:1043655. https://doi.org/10.3389/fnut.2022.1043655.

28 Mozaffari H, Hosseini Z, Lafrenière J, Conklin AI. The role of dietary diversity in preventing metabolic-related outcomes: findings from a systematic review. Obes Rev. 2021;22(6):e13174. https://doi.org/10.1111/obr.13174.

29 Rahman MM, de Silva A, Sassa M, Islam MR, Aktar S, Akter S. A systematic analysis and future projections of the nutritional status and interpretation of its drivers among school-aged children in South-East Asian countries. Lancet Reg Health Southeast Asia. 2023;16:100244. https://doi.org/10.1016/j.lansea.2023.100244.

30 Elizabeth KE. Infant and young child feeding—a panacea for current & future health with macro and micronutrient sufficiency. Ind J Pract Pediatr. 2023;25(1):43–8.

31 World Health Organization. Infant and young child feeding [cited 2024 Jan 27]. Available from: https://www.who.int/data/nutrition/nlis/info/infant-and-young-child-feeding.

32 FAO, IFAD, UNICEF, WFP, and WHO. The State of Food Security and Nutrition in the World 2023. Urbanization, Agrifood Systems Transformation and Healthy Diets Across the Rural–Urban Continuum. Rome: FAO; 2023. https://doi.org/10.4060/cc3017en.

33 Sun Strategy 3.0 [cited 2024 Jan 31]. Available from: https://scalingupnutrition.org/sites/default/files/2022-08/SUN-Strategy-2021-2025_ENG_web1.pdf.

George Jacob Elizabeth
Department of Pediatrics
Ananthapuri Hospitals & Research Institute
Chaka NH, Bypass
Thiruvananthapuram, Kerala 695024, India
drelizake@gmail.com

Published online: November 15, 2024

Szajewska H, Neu J, Shamir R, Wong G, Prentice AM (eds): Shaping the Future with Nutrition. Nestle Nutr Inst Workshop Ser. Basel, Karger, 2024, vol 100, pp 125–138 (DOI: 10.1159/000540143)

Two Sides of the Same Coin: Strategies to Address Under- and Over-Nutrition

Andrew M. Prentice

MRC Unit The Gambia at London School of Hygiene and Tropical Medicine, Banjul, The Gambia

Abstract

Although malnutrition in the form of child wasting, stunting, and micronutrient deficiencies remain prevalent on many of the poorest and war-torn places on earth, there has been major progress in other regions and the direction of travel remains generally good. However, as countries pass through the economic transition there has been a seemingly inevitable rise in overweight and obesity with its attendant personal health costs (reduced life span due to obesity-related chronic conditions) and a rise in the societal costs of care. Strategies, by healthcare professionals and others, to combat the two sides of the malnutrition coin must be built on a solid foundational knowledge of the causes of each condition. The individual, nutritional, and environmental drivers are summarized here. It is sometimes helpful to focus on a single unifying concept as a way of rationalizing the causes and required solutions; namely the nutrient density of foods. Malnutrition is caused, inter alia, by foods lacking in sufficient energy, protein, and micronutrients. The same is true for obesity which, in large part, is driven by foods overly dense in energy but lacking other critical nutrients. Food quality therefore emerges as a key concept that healthcare professionals can adopt as they educate parents and children at the microlevel and schools, health systems, and government bodies at the macrolevel.

Introduction

Global progress against most forms of undernutrition has been impressive in recent decades but this has been accompanied by a seemingly inexorable rise in overweight and obesity. There are very few countries worldwide that have managed to balance a low prevalence of undernutrition with low rates of overnutrition. This leads to the so-called double burden of malnutrition in many nations.

There are many drivers of these changes but the primary one is economic development (see Fig. 1). As countries progress through the economic transition anthropometric health metrics improve (stunting and wasting rates decline) but then start to deteriorate again (overweight and obesity rates climb). These reciprocal trends represent the "two sides of the same coin" discussed in this article.

In order to devise strategies to combat under- and over-nutrition it is first important to understand the nature of the problem and the factors that cause individuals and sub-populations to deviate from a healthy body size.

Etiological Drivers of Malnutrition

For the purposes of the current discussion, malnutrition is defined either as an abnormally low weight or height (wasting/stunting), or an abnormally high weight and fat mass (overweight/obesity).

The many possible drivers of these extremes are summarized in Figure 2. Ultimately any deviations in anthropometric status must be mediated through effects on an individual's physiology and metabolism depicted in the center of the graphic.

The calibration of a person's innate responses to energy and nutrients is strongly influenced by their genetic inheritance. This has been studied in greatest detail in relation to obesity, the propensity to which can be determined in very rare circumstances by monogenic defects, but much more generally by the inheritance of a cluster of common gene variants that each contribute a slight tendency towards weight gain. Genome-wide association studies have identified nearly one thousand obesity or fat mass risk variants [1]. Combination of these into a "polygenic risk score" provides a more holistic assessment of a person's genetic risk, but it is important to emphasize that these scores are not deterministic; they simply portray a tendency. For example, in a study of ~18,000 Swedish adults a one standard deviation difference in the polygenic risk score for obesity only accounted for a body mass index difference of 1.1 kg/m^2 in

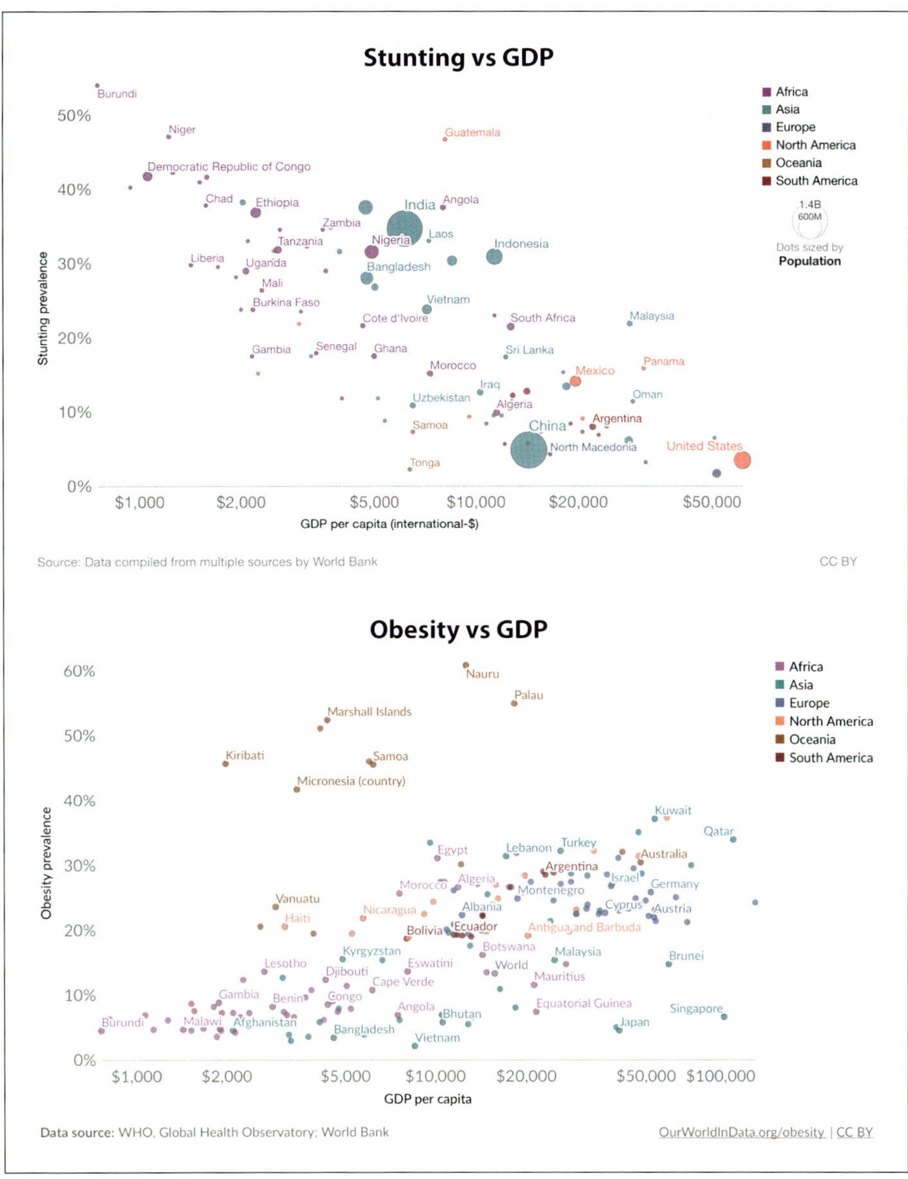

Fig. 1. Reciprocal relationships between under- and over-nutrition according to national gross domestic product (GDP). Data from WHO Global Health Observatory, World Bank and additional sources complied by OurWorldInData.org.

middle-aged adults [2]. The genetics of leanness has been little studied but the reciprocal of a polygenic risk score for obesity effectively represents a likelihood of being lean or underweight.

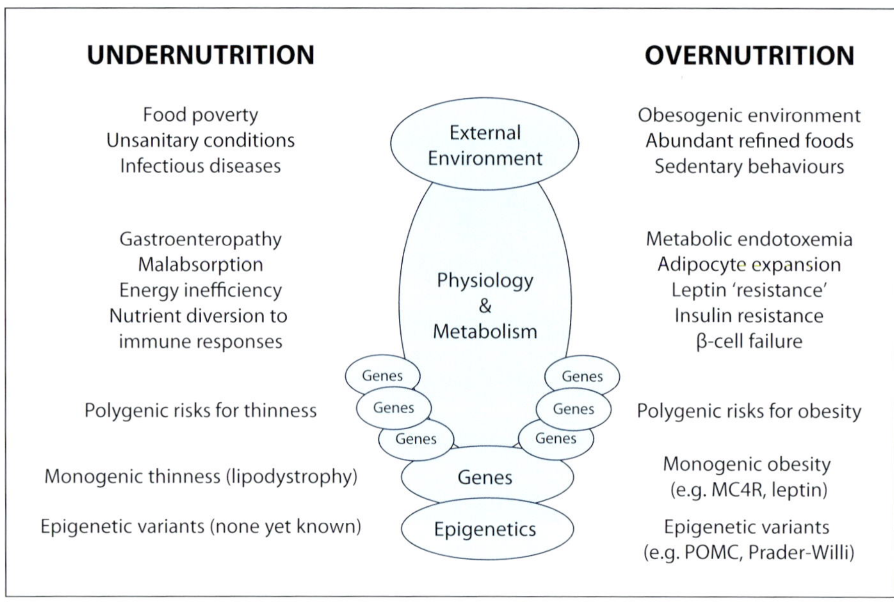

Fig. 2. Multilevel interactions leading to under- or over-nutrition.

Epigenetic variants can also influence a person's likelihood of being lean or obese. Some rare epigenetic defects (e.g., a failure of imprinting in Prader-Willi syndrome) cause severe obesity whilst other more common variations contribute to the likelihood of obesity. For instance, variable methylation in the promoter region of the *POMC* gene is associated with obesity [3]. Again, the reciprocal of an epigenetic risk for obesity is also equivalent to a tendency towards leanness.

The innate metabolism, molded by these genetic and epigenetic influences, interacts with external environmental influences. The effects of these are modulated by peoples' individual behaviors and choices. Table 1 lists some of the individual, nutritional, and environmental influences on stunting and wasting, and Table 2 lists the contrasting influences on overweight and obesity. The great majority of the multiple factors listed in these summaries are theoretically amenable to interventions.

Global Success in Reducing Under-Nutrition

There are still far too many stunted and underweight children in the world, as well as mothers and young children suffering from a range of micronutrient deficiencies (so-called "hidden hunger"). Nonetheless, progress towards the

Table 1. Individual and environmental factors causing stunting and/or wasting

Individual	Nutritional	Environmental
Genetic – small parental size, rare metabolic disorders **Intergenerational** – stunting in prior generations, epigenetic transmission **Poor fetal growth** – prematurity, low birthweight, stunting at birth **Physical abnormalities** – orofacial defects (e.g., cleft palate), cerebral palsy **Gut microbiome** – delayed maturation of microbiome **Parental** – poor parental understanding of childcare **Emotional** – e.g., child neglect/ abuse	**Breastfeeding** – poor establishment of breastfeeding, low milk volume in some mothers **Weaning foods** – dilute and contaminated first foods **Macronutrient deficiencies** – insufficient protein and energy **Micronutrient deficiencies** – deficiencies of Type 2 (growth affecting) micronutrients **Monotonous diets** – low palatability of many foods **Inappropriate foods** – energy rich, nutrient poor processed foods **Food allergies** – e.g., lactose intolerance, specific allergies	**Childhood infections** – especially gastrointestinal and respiratory infections **Gastroenteropathy** – persistent gut damage leads to malabsorption and nutrient leakage **Low grade inflammation** – inflammation blocks nutrient absorption and utilisation **Immune activation** – energy and nutrients are diverted to support immune responses **Helminth infections** – compete for nutrients **Heat** – suppresses appetite

Table 2. Individual and environmental factors causing overweight and obesity

Individual	Nutritional	Environmental
Genetic – inherited polygenic risks, rare monogenic causes **Epigenetic** – imprinting disorders, altered methylome **Intergenerational** – obesity in prior generations **Fetal overgrowth** – macrosomia, maternal obesity, gestational diabetes in the mother **Gut microbiome** – firmicutes dominant microbiome increases energy extraction **Parental** – poor parental understanding of childcare **Emotional** – e.g., child neglect/ abuse may lead to binge eating and other disorders	**Breastfeeding** – breastfeeding protects against obesity **Weaning foods** – inappropriate weaning foods including high-protein formulas **Excess energy density of diets** – humans have poor satiety responses **Ultra-extracted foodstuffs** – refined oils and sugars increase energy density **Sugar-sweetened beverages** – liquid calories are easily ingested in excess **Snacking and binge eating** – food always available at relatively low cost	**Obesogenic food environment** – see below **Cost of food** – cost of food has declined relative to disposable income **Marketing** – inappropriate promotions to children, marketing based on quantity not quality **Supersizing** – excessive portion sizes, eat-all-you-want and two-for-one marketing **Energy-sparing devices** – reduced cost of work, household activities and locomotion **Sedentary occupations** – office work **Sedentary leisure behaviours** – excess TV viewing, computer/ phone usage, gaming **Changing social norms** – obesity now more usual/acceptable, environment is permissive

elimination of malnutrition has been impressive. This achievement has been driven by national governments spurred on by the Millennium Development Goals and subsequent Sustainable Development Goals, with guidance from numerous non-governmental alliances.

Some of the progress has been achieved through the short-term strategies of supplementation programs; UNICEF's support of childhood vitamin A supplementation being a prime example. Other progress has been achieved through fortification; with iodine fortification of salt, vigorously and successfully promoted by the International Council for the Control of Iodine Deficiency Disorders working with UNICEF and WHO among others, making goiter and fetal abnormalities rare in the modern world.

Much of the progress has also been achieved through economic advancement and the ability of peoples to access foods with a higher nutrient density, many of them produced in large scale by local or multinational corporations. Manufactured foods have been a major driver of improved nutritional status globally, but can also contribute to ill health if eaten in excess; another aspect of the "two sides of the same coin" in the title of this presentation.

The improved nutritional status of children is not solely due to improved nutrition; there is an important contribution from improvements in hygiene and disease reduction. But even the combination of these so-called nutrition-specific and nutrition-sensitive measures struggles to have impact without the remaining holistic benefits that derive from economic advancement. The excellent WASH Benefits [4, 5] and SHINE Trials [6] provide a clear example of this. In these large well-executed randomized trials in Kenya, Bangladesh, and Zimbabwe education of mothers in the principles of Infant and Young Child Feeding achieved only a small improvement in stunting and the WASH hygiene interventions disappointingly achieved no benefit. The interpretation has been that the interventions were insufficiently robust and penetrant, leading to calls for "transformative WASH" [7] as indicated by our own research in rural Gambia in which we found evidence of a very high hygiene threshold before child growth normalizes [8]. Reference to Figure 1 indicates that a doubling of GDP results in approximately a one-third reduction in national stunting rates.

Strategies to Address the Double Burden of Malnutrition

Public health strategies to combat malnutrition can be considered among many domains from the macro scale downwards. Health systems, food systems, education, manufacturing, pricing, and taxation – all of which can be influenced by national government policies – can play a pivotal role. Sadly, however, as mentioned above, few countries have managed to optimize their population's nutritional status and prevent the pendulum swinging from undernutrition to overnutrition.

At a more granular level, parents necessarily have a huge role in determining their children's nutritional status, and in turn, they can derive advice from their healthcare professionals. This article will only discuss these aspects.

Strategies to Address Undernutrition

Life Course Influences

A very recent meta-analysis of almost 84,000 children from 33 longitudinal cohorts worldwide examined the influence of 30 different exposures as determinants of childhood wasting and stunting [9]. A key finding was that population improvements in maternal height and birth size would produce a substantial improvement in height-for-age and weight-for-age Z-scores at 24 months. In fact, these were the dominant determinants of child growth patterns up to 2 years of age, and far outweighed more proximal determinants such as exclusive breastfeeding to 6 months.

The take-home message from these and similar analyses is that once a baby has been conceived a substantial proportion of its growth trajectory can already be predicted on the basis of preceding exposures (genetics of mother and father), intergenerational effects [10], and nutrition during the mother's own life course [11]. These influences place upper limits on what can be achieved through pre- or post-natal interventions, but should not be construed as indicating that later intervention is futile. Rather than be fatalistic, parents and healthcare professionals should work to optimize the growth gains and associated health and developmental benefits that can be achieved.

Early Infant Feeding

Exclusive or predominant breastfeeding has many important, often lifesaving, benefits for newborns and their mothers [12]. However, it is not associated with protection against stunting though appears to be marginally protective against wasting [9, 13] and protects against obesity (see below).

In many populations, it is the transition from breastfeeding, through first weaning foods and towards a mature diet that is challenging. The much-cited analysis of growth data from 54 national surveys in low- and middle-income countries first published by Victora [14] makes this point very clear. Compared to the WHO 50th centile growth target, children were born small but grew very well in the first 3 months of life, before then falling away from the target for both weight and more so for height. It has been recognized for many decades that a key contributor to the growth faltering that often associates with the introduction of non-breastmilk foods is the very poor quality and bacterial contamination of first-weaning foods [15]. Feeding trials of young infants and children in Bangladesh have elegantly illustrated the huge importance of both energy/nutrient density of foods and feeding frequency in optimizing nutrient intakes [16].

Providing guidance for parents and healthcare professionals alike the World Health Organization has recently updated its guidance on Complementary

Feeding [17] which acts as buttress to WHO's earlier guidance on Infant and Young Child Feeding [18]. The key recommendations targeted at optimizing healthy growth and nutritional status are extracted in Figure 3.

Breastfeeding, preferably exclusively to 6 months if the mother has the capacity, is recommended to continue until 2 years or beyond (Recommendation 1). In practice, there are few cultures where breastfeeding beyond 2 years is common. Weaning foods should start to be introduced at 6 months (180 days) if not before (Recommendation 2). From 6 to 12 months, infants are recommended to have animal or animal-based formula milks and an increasing diversity of other foods with emphasis on daily consumption of animal-sourced foods, fruits and vegetables, and frequent consumption of pulses, nuts, and seeds if animal source foods are in poor supply (Recommendations 3&4). Recommendation 6 proposes that nutrient supplements and/or fortified foods can be useful when nutrient requirements cannot be met from unfortified foods alone. Recommendation 6b contains a perplexing and questionable statement that consumption of commercial cereal-based foods should not be encouraged, which runs counter to the fact that improvements in child growth in most modern societies have occurred in the presence of such products that have tailored nutritional content and are safely and hygienically packaged for point-of-use feeding to toddlers.

Transitions to the Childhood and Adult Diet

As children's ability to digest and metabolize complex foods with a high solute load matures the child can be increasingly exposed to the normal adult diet. In communities that eat from shared bowls, it is important to ensure that the young child is allowed its share and is given sufficient time to eat to satiety. More frequent feeding is also desirable, especially if the adult diet has a low energy and nutrient density.

As in younger infants, the need for a high nutrient (especially protein) density and frequent feeding is especially critical after episodes of illness that have caused growth faltering and weight loss.

Environmental Influences

As summarized in Table 1 there are many powerful environmental influences that inhibit child growth in poor environments. Childhood infections, especially gastrointestinal and respiratory infections, have acute effects through inhibition of appetite as well as the catabolic effects of immune activation where nutrients and energy are diverted to support immune defenses.

There are additional longer-term effects. Low-grade inflammation is almost universal in children living in less hygienic conditions and this blocks nutrient

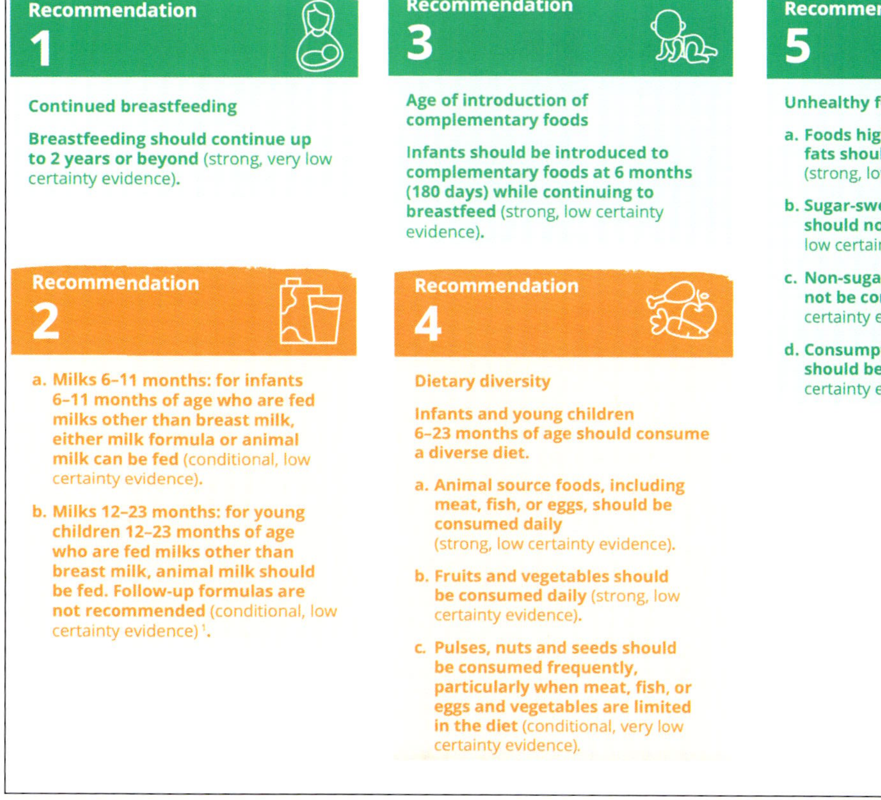

Fig. 3. Latest WHO recommendations on Infant and Young Child Feeding (IYCF). Reproduced with permission from WHO Guideline for complementary feeding of infants and young children 6–23 months of age. Switzerland. World Health Organization; 2023. Licence: CC BY-NC-SA 3.0 IGO.

absorption and utilization [19]; the effect on iron absorption mediated by the iron-regulating hormone hepcidin is especially pronounced [20]. Gastroenteropathy, a persistent gut damage often termed "environmental enteric disease", leads to malabsorption and nutrient leakage through villous atrophy and leaks in the gut epithelium [21]. Furthermore, helminth infections, where present, compete for nutrients, and high temperatures can suppress appetite. Aflatoxin exposure, common in many rural communities in hot environments, is also associated with stunting [22].

Finally, there is evidence that the gut microbiome fails to mature at the appropriate post-natal rate in malnourished children and this may be an additional risk factor (or consequence) of growth failure [23] leading to calls for microbiota-directed therapeutic foods [24].

As mentioned above, it would be logical to conclude that WASH interventions should greatly improve child growth but these have, so far, had disappointing outcomes at the population level and point to the need for much more effective intervention in the form of "transformative WASH". This should not discourage healthcare professionals from educating parents that their children's growth will be impaired by unhygienic living conditions.

Strategies to Address Overnutrition and Obesity

Life Course Influences

Excluding the influence of genetics there are many ways that obesity can be transmitted from generation to generation [25]. Overweight and obese mothers are considerably more likely to give birth to a macrosomic baby that already carries an extra risk of later-life obesity [26]. Primarily, parental influences can be transmitted through shared dietary and exercise habits which are theoretically amenable to intervention, but in practice require very significant educational and motivational inputs by healthcare professionals. Most parents are generally aware of the dangers of obesity to their children and of the general principles of healthy lifestyles, but putting knowledge into practice is very challenging.

Early Infant Feeding

There is evidence that breastfeeding protects children from obesity, though, as with all association studies of breastfeeding, adjustment for confounding is challenging (breastfeeding mothers tend to be better educated and healthier) but the protective effect nonetheless appears to be real [27].

Old-style infant formulas also led to higher adiposity in infants but decades of development designed to better mimic the nutritional attributes of human milk (especially by lowering the protein content) have reduced this difference [28].

Parental desire to have an infant that fulfills the advertised stereotype that associates plumpness with good health and happiness can easily lead to overfeeding especially in a bottle-fed baby. Assisting parents to overcome the misplaced association between an overweight baby and a healthy baby represents an important role played by healthcare professionals. Education of parents in the skills of "responsive feeding" is a useful intervention at this stage.

Transitions to the Childhood Diet

The time at which toddlers transition towards a childhood and then adult diet is a critical risk period for obesity. Parents limited by finance, time, and education can easily allow their children to start consuming a "junk" diet with an excess of highly energy-dense fast foods and sugar-sweetened beverages. Excess consumption of fruit juices is also a risk even though fruit juice may be perceived as healthy.

Environmental Influences

The term "*Obesogenic Environment*" was coined to draw together the numerous changes that have coalesced over the past 50 or so years to create conditions that are highly favorable to the development of obesity – in short, gluttony and sloth [29]. But whilst gluttony and sloth were amongst the original deadly sins, modern children are innocent of such blame and instead have become victims to their external environment.

On the intake side of the energy balance equation, the cost of food (calories) has generally declined as a proportion of disposable income for all but the poorest people on earth. Marketers, particularly of foods for people on a small budget, have used quantity in place of quality as a marketing ploy. Supersizing is rife [30], portion sizes are often excessive, and eat-all-you-want and two-for-one offers are commonplace. In many countries, there are inappropriate promotions of energy-dense snacks and junk foods to children.

Energy expenditure has also greatly declined [31]. For adults this comes in the form of major reductions in the energy cost of manual work (through the use of mechanical tools), of transport and locomotion (through increasing use of cars, e-bikes, elevators, escalators, travelators, etc.), and of household activities (through increasing number of energy-sparing gadgets for home and garden). Increasing proportions have sedentary work in offices. Some of these changes affect children; for instance, increasing numbers are taken to and from school by car (often due to safety concerns in the built environment).

There has also been large-scale adoption of sedentary leisure behaviors in the form of (often excessive) TV viewing, computer and phone usage, and gaming; the latter of which can affect even very young children.

Finally, in many countries, there has been a profound change in social norms such that obesity is now more usual and acceptable, and the physical environment is being re-engineered in ways that are permissive towards obesity. In many ways these changes are to be highly welcomed insofar as they temper what was previously a very high level of prejudice, but they do remove one corrective brake and thus make obesity even more common.

Strategies to combat childhood overweight and obesity require a holistic approach with efforts at all levels of society from family to local and national government [31]. Education as to the huge health risks and costs that accompany obesity at both the individual and societal level are the starting point, and this is where healthcare professionals can and should play a leading role.

A Unifying Concept That Links the Two Sides of the Malnutrition Coin

Nutrient density is a key determinant of nutritional health. Many traditional diets, and particularly traditional weaning foods for infants and toddlers in low-income settings, have very low nutrient density (energy, protein, and micronutrients) and hence have been associated with poor growth. Carefully balanced alternatives have been manufactured and have driven the improvements in growth in most advanced nations, but remain unaffordable for most of the world. Unfortunately, this gap has been filled by ultra-processed "junk" foods which have high energy levels of refined energy (sugars, fats, and sodium) but lack fiber and quality micronutrients. Energy density is a major driver of weight gain and adiposity [32]. Families with a poor understanding of the principles of nutrition allow their children to consume excess amounts of such foods with inevitable consequences; weight gain, obesity, and associated metabolic diseases. Of note recent research suggests that, as yet unknown, aspects of "ultra" processing of foods contribute to poor heart health and diabetes [e.g., 33].

The EAT-Lancet recommendations for diets in the Anthropocene make cogent suggestions as to how families should modify their food plate to optimize their own as well as the planet's health [34]. Unfortunately, their application would require levels of nutritional education well beyond most people. A return to more traditional, unrefined, and locally grown foods is an admirable goal but, unless accompanied by a sophisticated understanding of the principles of good nutrition – especially good child nutrition – may lead to a resurgence in nutrient deficiencies. Thus, food manufacturers will continue to play a vital role in feeding the planet. As the dangers of excess energy density and low nutrient content of "junk" foods becomes ever more obvious, and the concerns of ultra-processing start to be understood, responsible manufacturers will find fertile markets within populations whose nutritional awareness is gradually becoming more sophisticated.

Conflict of Interest Statement

The author received travel support to attend NNIW100 and an honorarium from NNI for preparing this paper. He is a member of the Global Nestlé Nutrition Institute Scientific Council.

References

1 Yengo L, Sidorenko J, Kemper KE, Zheng Z, Wood AR, Weedon MN, et al. Meta-analysis of genome-wide association studies for height and body mass index in ~700000 individuals of European ancestry. Hum Mol Genet. 2018;27(20):3641–9. https://doi.org/10.1093/hmg/ddy271

2 Ojalehto E, Zhan Y, Jylhävä J, Reynolds CA, Dahl Aslan AK, Karlsson IK. Genetically and environmentally predicted obesity in relation to cardiovascular disease: a nationwide cohort study. EClinicalMedicine. 2023;58:101943. https://doi.org/10.1016/j.eclinm.2023.101943

3 Lechner L, Opitz R, Silver MJ, Krabusch PM, Prentice AM, Field MS, et al. Early-set POMC methylation variability is accompanied by increased risk for obesity and is addressable by MC4R agonist treatment. Sci Transl Med. 2023;15(705):eadg1659. https://doi.org/10.1126/scitranslmed.adg1659

4 Null C, Stewart CP, Pickering AJ, Dentz HN, Arnold BF, Arnold CD, et al. Effects of water quality, sanitation, handwashing, and nutritional interventions on diarrhoea and child growth in rural Kenya: a cluster-randomised controlled trial. Lancet Glob Health. 2018;6(3):e316–29. https://doi.org/10.1016/S2214-109X(18)30005-6

5 Luby SP, Rahman M, Arnold BF, Unicomb L, Ashraf S, Winch PJ, et al. Effects of water quality, sanitation, handwashing, and nutritional interventions on diarrhoea and child growth in rural Bangladesh: a cluster randomised controlled trial. Lancet Glob Health. 2018;6(3):e302–15. https://doi.org/10.1016/S2214-109X(17)30490-4

6 Humphrey JH, Mbuya MNN, Ntozini R, Moulton LH, Stoltzfus RJ, Tavengwa NV, et al. Independent and combined effects of improved water, sanitation, and hygiene, and improved complementary feeding, on child stunting and anaemia in rural Zimbabwe: a cluster-randomised trial. Lancet Glob Health. 2019;7(1):e132–47. https://doi.org/10.1016/S2214-109X(18)30374-7

7 Cumming O, Arnold BF, Ban R, Clasen T, Esteves Mills J, Freeman MC, et al. The implications of three major new trials for the effect of water, sanitation and hygiene on childhood diarrhea and stunting: a consensus statement. BMC Med. 2019;17(1):173. https://doi.org/10.1186/s12916-019-1410-x

8 Husseini M, Darboe MK, Moore SE, Nabwera HM, Prentice AM. Thresholds of socio-economic and environmental conditions necessary to escape from childhood malnutrition: a natural experiment in rural Gambia. BMC Med. 2018;16(1):199. https://doi.org/10.1186/s12916-018-1179-3

9 Mertens A, Benjamin-Chung J, Colford JM Jr, Coyle J, van der Laan MJ, Hubbard AE, et al. Causes and consequences of child growth faltering in low-resource settings. Nature. 2023;621(7979):568–76. https://doi.org/10.1038/s41586-023-06501-x

10 Eriksen KG, Radford EJ, Silver MJ, Fulford AJC, Wegmüller R, Prentice AM. Influence of intergenerational *in utero* parental energy and nutrient restriction on offspring growth in rural Gambia. FASEB J. 2017;31(11):4928–34. https://doi.org/10.1096/fj.201700017R

11 Fleming TP, Watkins AJ, Velazquez MA, Mathers JC, Prentice AM, Stephenson J, et al. Origins of lifetime health around the time of conception: causes and consequences. Lancet. 2018;391(10132):1842–52. https://doi.org/10.1016/S0140-6736(18)30312-X

12 Victora CG, Bahl R, Barros AJD, França GVA, Horton S, Krasevec J, et al. Breastfeeding in the 21st century: epidemiology, mechanisms, and lifelong effect. Lancet. 2016;387(10017):475–90. https://doi.org/10.1016/S0140-6736(15)01024-7

13 Giugliani ERJ, Horta BL, Loret de Mola C, Lisboa BO, Victora CG. Effect of breastfeeding promotion interventions on child growth: a systematic review

and meta-analysis. Acta Paediatr. 2015;104(467): 20–9. https://doi.org/10.1111/apa.13160

14 Victora CG, de Onis M, Hallal PC, Blössner M, Shrimpton R. Worldwide timing of growth faltering: revisiting implications for interventions. Pediatrics. 2010;125(3):e473–80. https://doi.org/10.1542/peds.2009-1519

15 Rowland MG, Barrell RA, Whitehead RG. Bacterial contamination in traditional Gambian weaning foods. Lancet. 1978;1(8056):136–8. https://doi.org/10.1016/s0140-6736(78)90432-4

16 Islam MM, Khatun M, Peerson JM, Ahmed T, Mollah MA, Dewey KG, et al. Effects of energy density and feeding frequency of complementary foods on total daily energy intakes and consumption of breast milk by healthy breastfed Bangladeshi children. Am J Clin Nutr. 2008;88(1): 84–94. https://doi.org/10.1093/ajcn/88.1.84

17 WHO Guideline for Complementary Feeding of Infants and Young Children 6–23 Months of Age. Geneva: World Health Organization; 2023.

18 WHO. Global Strategy for Infant and Young Child Feeding. Geneva: World Health Organisation; 2023.

19 Prendergast AJ, Rukobo S, Chasekwa B, Mutasa K, Ntozini R, Mbuya MN, et al. Stunting is characterized by chronic inflammation in Zimbabwean infants. PLoS One. 2014;9(2):e86928. https://doi.org/10.1371/journal.pone.0086928

20 Prentice AM, Bah A, Jallow MW, Jallow AT, Sanyang S, Sise EA, et al. Respiratory infections drive hepcidin-mediated blockade of iron absorption leading to iron deficiency anemia in African children. Sci Adv. 2019;5(3):eaav9020. https://doi.org/10.1126/sciadv.aav9020

21 Humphrey JH. Child undernutrition, tropical enteropathy, toilets, and handwashing. Lancet. 2009;374(9694):1032–5. https://doi.org/10.1016/S0140-6736(09)60950-8

22 Watson S, Moore SE, Darboe MK, Chen G, Tu YK, Huang YT, et al. Impaired growth in rural Gambian infants exposed to aflatoxin: a prospective cohort study. BMC Publ Health. 2018;18(1):1247. https://doi.org/10.1186/s12889-018-6164-4

23 Subramanian S, Huq S, Yatsunenko T, Haque R, Mahfuz M, Alam MA, et al. Persistent gut microbiota immaturity in malnourished Bangladeshi children. Nature. 2014;510(7505):417–21. https://doi.org/10.1038/nature13421

24 Blanton LV, Barratt MJ, Charbonneau MR, Ahmed T, Gordon JI. Childhood undernutrition, the gut microbiota, and microbiota-directed therapeutics. Science. 2016;352(6293):1533. https://doi.org/10.1126/science.aad9359

25 Comas-Armangue G, Makharadze L, Gomez-Velazquez M, Teperino R. The legacy of parental obesity: mechanisms of non-genetic transmission and reversibility. Biomedicines. 2022;10:2461. https://doi.org/10.3390/biomedicines10102461

26 Hammoud NM, Visser GHA, van Rossem L, Biesma DH, Wit JM, de Valk HW. Long-term BMI and growth profiles in offspring of women with gestational diabetes. Diabetologia. 2018;61(5):1037–45. https://doi.org/10.1007/s00125-018-4584-4

27 Horta BL, Rollins N, Dias MS, Garcez V, Pérez-Escamilla R. Systematic review and meta-analysis of breastfeeding and later overweight or obesity expands on previous study for World Health Organization. Acta Paediatr. 2023;112(1):34–41. https://doi.org/10.1111/apa.16460

28 Koletzko B, Demmelmair H, Grote V, Totzauer M. Optimized protein intakes in term infants support physiological growth and promote long-term health. Semin Perinatol. 2019;43(7):151153. https://doi.org/10.1053/j.semperi.2019.06.001

29 Prentice AM, Jebb SA. Obesity in Britain: gluttony or sloth? BMJ. 1995;311(7002):437–9. https://doi.org/10.1136/bmj.311.7002.437

30 Rolls BJ. The supersizing of America: portion size and the obesity epidemic. Nutr Today. 2003;38(2): 42–53. https://doi.org/10.1097/00017285-200303000-00004

31 Swinburn BA, Sacks G, Hall KD, McPherson K, Finegood DT, Moodie ML, et al. The global obesity pandemic: shaped by global drivers and local environments. Lancet. 2011;378(9793):804–14. https://doi.org/10.1016/S0140-6736(11)60813-1

32 Prentice AM, Jebb SA. Fast foods, energydensity and obesity: a possible mechanistic link. Obes Rev. 2003;4:187–94. https://doi.org/10.1046/j.1467-789x.2003.00117.x

33 Wang L, Pan XF, Munro HM, Shrubsole MJ, Yu D. Consumption of ultra-processed foods and all-cause and cause-specific mortality in the Southern Community Cohort Study. Clin Nutr. 2023;42(10):1866–74. https://doi.org/10.1016/j.clnu.2023.08.012

34 Willett W, Rockström J, Loken B, Springmann M, Lang T, Vermeulen S, et al. Food in the Anthropocene: the EAT-Lancet Commission on healthy diets from sustainable food systems. Lancet. 2019;393(10170):447–92. https://doi.org/10.1016/S0140-6736(18)31788-4

Andrew M. Prentice
Head, Nutrition & Planetary Health
MRC Unit The Gambia at London School of Hygiene and Tropical Medicine
Atlantic Boulevard
Fajara, Banjul, The Gambia
andrew.prentice@lshtm.ac.uk

Published online: November 15, 2024

Szajewska H, Neu J, Shamir R, Wong G, Prentice AM (eds): Shaping the Future with Nutrition. Nestle Nutr Inst Workshop Ser. Basel, Karger, 2024, vol 100, pp 139–149 (DOI: 10.1159/000540144)

What Does Healthy Microbiome Development Look Like? State of the Art and Beyond

Giles Major[a, b, c] Shaillay Kumar Dogra[a]
Norbert Sprenger[a]

[a]Nestlé Institute of Health Sciences, Nestlé Research, Société des Produits Nestlé, Lausanne, Switzerland; [b]Nottingham NIHR Biomedical Research Centre, School of Medicine, University of Nottingham, Nottingham, UK; [c]Clinical Nutrition, Service d'Endocrinologie, Diabétologie et Métabolisme, Centre Hospitalier Universitaire Vaudoise (CHUV), Lausanne, Switzerland

Abstract

The community of microorganisms colonizing the gut changes during the first postnatal years of life. This ecosystem, henceforth described as the microbiome, modulates infant physiology and health, but uncertainty remains about the significance of variation in microbiome composition and function. Some may be tolerable, yet some microbiomes may be less healthy than others. Most efforts to identify parameters of microbiome health focus on adults, and derived concepts may not directly translate to early life that is characterized by dynamic and sequential changes. Data suggest that an orderly progression from an immature neonatal microbiome to a mature adult state is preferable to delayed or over-rapid development. This can be parameterized as a "microbiome development trajectory". Diet modifies early life microbiome development and is the principal modifiable factor to this end. Infants fed with infant formulas show different microbiome development trajectories from breastfed infants. Early data suggest that formulas containing a specific blend of human milk oligosaccharides partially mitigate this difference. Introduction of a complementary diet complexifies the identification of diet-microbiome development interactions. A better understanding will only be achievable through detailed, longitudinal characterization of large cohorts.

Introduction

125 years ago George Bernard Shaw wrote "The Doctor's Dilemma" in which he satirized a surgeon who believed that all health problems arose from a 'miasma in the colon' and could be relieved by colectomy. Scientific understanding of the relationship between the gut microbiome and health has progressed significantly since but many myths and misconceptions remain [1]. One area of confident consensus is that the gut microbiome changes rapidly in human early postnatal life [2]. Since early structure may direct later stable composition of the microbial community in the gut, it is relevant to consider whether variations in microbiome development matter and what can be done about them. This chapter explores our current understanding of the roles of the gut microbiome; methods by which to characterize it; the necessary modifications to these principles when considering early life; and the current state of knowledge on the capacity of diet to influence microbiome development towards a more stable and resilient mature state.

The Role of the Gut Microbiome

The existence of symbiotic relationships between bacteria and other kingdoms of life, such as animals and plants, is well established. From an evolutionary perspective, such relationships endure when there is mutual benefit: bacteria colonize an environmental niche and flourish; the "host" then derives additional benefit from the bacterial community.

The ecosystems that develop in these environmental niches are referred to as "microbiomes", capturing both the microbiota (archaea, fungi, bacteria, and protists) present together with their structural elements and activity in a distinct environment with its conditions, like the human gut for example [3]. It should be noted that the gut virome may also play a role in these ecological interactions [4]. Five hundred million years ago the evolution of the bilaterian gut, with separate points of entry (mouth) and exit (anus) as part of a polar body structure, created a novel niche to exploit. The "gut microbiome" has thus co-evolved with the gut, creating complementary functions for mutual advantage. For the host, the key roles of the gut include nutrient harvest, defense, and flow – both of material and information.

The key role of the gut is nutrient harvest: to convert complex molecules, such as proteins, fats, and carbohydrates, into simpler structures that can be absorbed and utilized for energy, function, and growth. The enzymes expressed by bacteria [5] complement the gut's digestive capacity from brush border enzymes and secretions from saliva and pancreatic juice to increase the breakdown of ingesta and so bioaccessibility of nutrients.

Two classic microbiome studies illustrate this. Firstly, Smith et al. showed that Malawian twins with different degrees of malnutrition harbored different microbiota, such that the twin with increased capacity to break down the fiber-rich Malawian diet was protected. Fecal transplant studies using gnotobiotic mice showed that this digestive trait could be transferred solely with the microbiota [6]. The gnotobiotic mouse model approach was also used by Turnbaugh et al. to show that the microbiota of obese mice could increase energy harvest in lean recipients [7].

The gut microbiome is also recognized to synthesize vitamins and may improve recovery of dietary minerals but illustrating such an effect is harder, particularly in the clinical setting where supplements can and should be used to offset the risks of deficiency. While the gnotobiotic animal model approach to prove causality is powerful, there are few scenarios where it can be used in humans. This leaves clinical microbiome studies open to the challenge that any effect is due to confounding, microbiome-independent pathways.

One scenario where confidence in causality can be found is the use of bacteriotherapy to treat recurrent diarrhea associated with *Clostridioides difficile*. The study by van Nood et al. that achieved 93% successful resolution with a nasogastric fecal microbial transplant protocol [8] stimulated a huge growth in the field most recently illustrated by the capability of live purified Firmicutes spores to improve recovery compared to antibiotic treatment [9]. Associated changes in colonic bile acid profiles illustrate how the microbiome supports pathogen suppression in the gut.

The microbiome also supports the immune response through production of modulating metabolites such as short-chain fatty acids and aromatic amino acid-derived indoles [10]. These circulating factors modulate inflammatory responses beyond the gut, so-called "axes" between the gut and skin, lung, or other organs [11]. Signaling through other means such as gut hormones or the enteric nervous system allows the microbiome to influence the transit of material through the gut. There is mounting evidence that this coordinating role extends to the central nervous system. Microbiome effects have been implicated in appetite, mood, and behavior, all of which remain consistent with the aim of the symbiotic host-microbiome relationship to maintain a healthy supply of nutrition for both bacteria and host.

Microbiome Development: Concept and Measurement

While there is a clear potential to harness the microbiome to improve health, it remains challenging to demonstrate health impact outside extreme situations such as microbiota transfer studies in gnotobiotic mice or patients with recurrent *C. difficile* infection. An alternative approach aims to use large-scale epidemiology to identify associations between microbiome features and health outcomes, then investigate potential mechanisms in the laboratory (bedside to bench) to develop microbiome modulators for application in clinical trials (bench to bedside). This cycle necessitates definition of candidate microbiome features (parameters) that may drive outcomes.

Microbiome parameters can be described with regard to two axes: whether they describe specific components of the microbiome or the whole ecosystem; and whether they describe microbiome composition or behavior (Table 1). Specific components of composition include key species or clades such as the *Bifidobacteria* [12], while ecosystem composition may be expressed as diversity – the number of different clades present and their relative proportions in the whole population. Specific elements of behavior include the profile of produced microbial metabolites, such as short-chain fatty acids, while an example of ecosystem behavior would be microbiome resilience [13]: the degree to which the community resists disruption (e.g., by antibiotics) and recovers to its former state. Some of these concepts may be in tension – the dominance of a particular clade of bacteria may reduce overall diversity – so it is important to establish how different parameters associate with health at different life stages.

Having established the conceptual challenges of microbiome measurement, it is important to appreciate the technical challenges. Recent advances in microbiome science have been driven by non-culture-based characterization: the identification of key nucleotide sequences through either quantitative amplification or next-generation sequencing. As described in the previous paragraph, there is also a balance between measuring composition and function.

Bacterial sequences can be compared to open catalogs of bacterial genomes to define the "operational taxonomic units" (akin to species) present. This creates a "map" of the bacteria present with possible function attributed according to prior knowledge. Alternatively, the composite genome of all the microbiota present – the metagenome – can be characterized directly according to present gene functions. While these data can be mapped to species or strains, as "metagenome-assembled genomes", the purpose of the method is to evaluate the functional capacity of the microbiome – the "guidebook" rather than the "map".

Table 1. Microbiome measures with a brief description of their meaning and key examples illustrating their association to infant health outcomes

Microbiota measure	Brief Description	Key examples
Alpha-diversity (Species richness, Shannon Index, Faith's Phylogenetic Diversity)	Indicates the overall complexity of the gut microbial ecosystem	Alpha-diversity was found to be lower for children who subsequently developed Type1 Diabetes [30] or Atopic disease [25]
Bacteria characterized at different taxonomic level	Captures key taxa	Bifidobacteria are a beneficial Genus for infants [11] *Bifidobacterium longum* subspecies *infantis* associated with protection against respiratory infections [31]
Beta-diversity	A distance measure of microbiota composition in comparison to another state, e.g., a reference or baseline	A shift closer to the breast-fed reference was demonstrated in an intervention trial with a blend of 5 HMOs [32] Subsequent cumulative asthma risk was higher for C-section born, if their microbiota was still dysbiotic compared to vaginally-delivered, at 1 year of age [23]
Microbiota age	An index to capture age-appropriate microbiota development	An aberrant microbiota age was reported for malnourished [32], atopic dermatitis [25], pediatric allergies [28] and autism spectrum disorder [33] children
Microbiota cluster types	Overall compositional states of microbiota communities	Progression to a particular cluster type associated with delivery mode, gestational duration and subsequent adiposity [34] A specific cluster type associated with reduced Antibiotics usage [35]
Networks of bacteria	Captures inter-relation of bacteria through their co-abundance network over time	Characterized healthy infant gut microbiota development that was distinct for the malnourished [36]
Functionality of the gut microbiome	Metabolites produced by the gut microbiome (e.g., short chain fatty acid, aromatic acid derived indoles, etc.)	Inverse association of butyrate, and bacteria with butyrate production potential, with asthma [29] and depletion in atopic eczema [37] At 3 months of age, association of acetate [31] and increased gamma-glutamylation and acetylation of amino-acids [38] with later protection from respiratory infections

Such advanced methods give greater granularity and coverage of the microbiome but also carry disadvantages: they report relative proportions of bacteria or genes, rather than absolute quantification, and cannot directly demonstrate bacterial function within the ecosystem. Other "-omics" approaches are needed to assess to what extent the functional capacity of the microbiome is translated into actual function. Targeted and untargeted metabolite profiling (metabolomics) are increasingly employed to this end. Further heterogeneity in technical aspects such as data annotation and analysis pipelines indicates that microbiome science remains a discipline requiring expertise, or at least caution about the limitations of "plug and play" approaches.

Microbiome Development: Factors Affecting Microbiome Development

Appreciation of the conceptual and technical elements of microbiome health science makes it easier to then consider the situation of early life when the gut microbiome develops rapidly and dynamically in infants and toddlers, [2, 14] and deviation from "normal" gut microbiome development may represent a risk for later health conditions (Fig. 1a). At around 2 to 3 years of age, the gut microbiome development will generally reach a more stable adult-like state. The main factors considered to enhance the microbiome's natural progression are vaginal delivery and exclusive breastfeeding for about 6 months followed by gradual introduction of solid food with continued breastfeeding up to 2 years [14]. Children following such criteria and developing normally may be considered suitable to establish a reference microbiome development trajectory.

Many factors have been shown to influence the natural succession and progression of the gut microbiome in early life. Among those are medical factors, like preterm- or C-section birth, and use of medications (in particular, antibiotics [16]). Additional microbiome changes are reported with numerous demographic factors like older siblings [17, 18] or furry pets [19] at home, geographical environment [20, 21], ethnicity [22], or cultural practices [23], for some likely due to variation in feeding practices.

Machine learning-based selection methods can help identify relevant microbiome features to describe normal gut microbiome development. One such approach is to select infant age discriminant features. This proved to be a promising approach allowing differentiation of microbiome development by different feeding modes for example [15] (Fig. 1b).

Few studies, using the microbiome development described through age-discriminant taxa, uncovered associations with later health condition. For

---

Fig. 1. a Schematic illustration of the gut microbiome development and main factors affecting it. To describe the gut microbiome development different metrics may be used like diversity measures, taxa, functions, or age discriminant taxa as shown in **b**. Red arrows indicate deviations from the normal development trajectory and green arrows indicate reversal of deviations. The differently colored bacteria indicate different taxa or functions of the gut microbiome. **b** A gut microbiota age model derived from the reference set obtained from the BCP-e cohort [39] (gestational age: >272 days, delivery method: vaginal, 4-month feeding ratio: exclusively breastfed, no antibiotics use, and weight-for-height z-score: >–3 and <3). Exclusive breastfed infants (n = 56 with 166 samples) represent the reference. Predominantly breastfed infants mostly breastmilk at 4 months (n = 10 with 29 samples). Formula fed infants were exclusively formula or more formula fed at 4 months (n = 11 with 21 samples). Microbiome development trajectory curves were fit using LOESS for data per feeding group and shaded regions depict 95% confidence intervals for these fits per group.

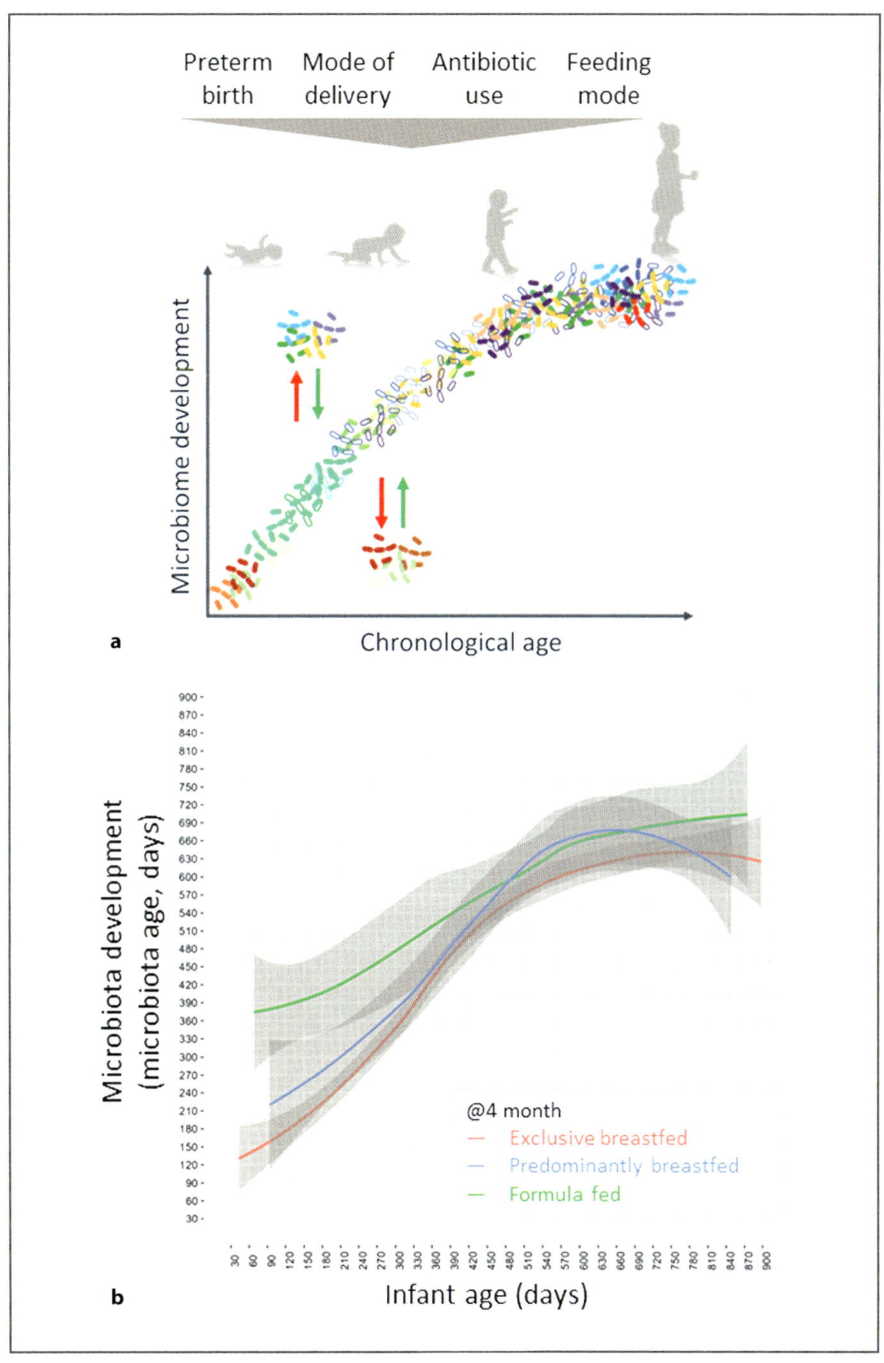
Preterm birth
Mode of delivery
Antibiotic use
Feeding mode
Microbiome development
Chronological age
a
Microbiota development (microbiota age, days)
900
870
840
810
780
750
720
690
660
630
600
570
540
510
480
450
420
390
360
330
300
270
240
210
180
150
120
90
60
30
@4 month
Exclusive breastfed
Predominantly breastfed
Formula fed
30 60 90 120 150 180 210 240 270 300 330 360 390 420 450 480 510 540 570 600 630 660 690 720 750 780 810 840 870 900
Infant age (days)
b

example, Galazzo et al. showed that a microbiome development progressing too fast early and too slow later in infants associated with later atopic dermatitis compared to healthy controls [25].

Dietary Manipulation to Optimize Microbiome Development

The gut microbiome is generally malleable by diet. Conceptually, any dietary component that escapes digestion in the upper gut may reach and affect the gut microbiome in the lower gut. Among those components, dietary non-digestible carbohydrates or fibers are key. With human milk being naturally the first and recommended diet in infancy, the human milk oligosaccharides (HMOs) being non-digestible fall within this group of microbiome-active components. Although HMOs are known to act on the gut microbiome for decades, they are increasingly recognized as key elements driving the early gut microbiome development mainly through specific infant-type bifidobacteria capable of metabolizing HMOs. In a recent trial with formula-fed infants, the addition of a specific blend of 5-HMOs drove the gut microbiome closer to that observed for vaginal-born breastfed infants both by using a global composition (beta-diversity) [26] and microbiome development trajectory measure. With the introduction of complementary diet, the early milk-oriented gut microbiome shifts increasingly towards a plant fiber-oriented microbiome. Likely, this transition in the gut microbiome is mediated by specific strains capable of metabolizing both HMOs and fibers like the recently described novel *Bifidobacterium longum* subspecies *iuvenis* [27]. Relatively little is known as to what specific dietary fibers are most age-adapted and relevant at the transition to family food [14]. Noteworthily, diet and fiber intake diversity become increasingly important as the microbiome reaches a more stable state, both in terms of establishing a diverse and resilient microbiome at around 2 to 3 years of age.

Microbiome Development and Its Link to Infant Development and Health

Early life microbiome establishment and progression assessed through different measures have been associated with several health outcomes, mostly related to immunity (Table 1). Infants born by C-section generally show gut microbial dysbiosis, like delayed bifidobacteria establishment, during the first postnatal months and were found to be associated with an increased risk to experience later asthma compared to vaginal-born infants [24]. In other studies, altered microbiome development, too fast or delayed, was associated in several studies to later pediatric allergy manifestations from atopic dermatitis to asthma [25, 28, 29].

These data underscore the need to understand the role of age-appropriate gut microbiome development. Just as for infant growth velocity, the orderly and timely development trajectory of the gut microbiome seems critical.

Constraints remain on our ability to link diet-mediated effects on the microbiome with healthy development. One such constraint is the lack of datasets that combine detailed dietary intake data with a dense frequency of microbiome sampling, adequate duration of follow-up, and a sufficient sample size to collect numerous health events.

Conclusion

The early life gut microbiome develops sequentially undergoing several presumably health-relevant phases. Advances in analytics allowed for ever-increasing insight in compositional and functional details of the gut microbiome. Advances in machine learning and data science allow grouping and filtering the sheer mass of data into interpretable portions. The combination of these techniques provides increasing insight into gut microbiome features that seem relevant for healthy infant development. Still, many aspects are only understood superficially when it comes to the interaction of different microbes at different stages of development and how these microbial networks and their metabolic activity affect infant development through a constant and bi-directional crosstalk.

Conflict of Interest Statement

All authors were employees of Société des Produits Nestlé S.A. at the time of authorship.

Author Contributions

G.M., S.K.D, and N.S. conceived the chapter. All authors contributed to the development of the chapter structure and content.

References

1 Walker AW, Hoyles L. Human microbiome myths and misconceptions. Nat Microbiol. 2023;8(8): 1392–6. https://doi.org/10.1038/s41564-023-01426-7.

2 Roswall J, Olsson LM, Kovatcheva-Datchary P, Nilsson S, Tremaroli V, Simon MC, et al. Developmental trajectory of the healthy human gut microbiota during the first 5 years of life. Cell Host

Microbe. 2021;29(5):765–76.e3. https://doi.org/10.1016/j.chom.2021.02.021.

3 Berg G, Rybakova D, Fischer D, Cernava T, Vergès MCC, Charles T, et al. Microbiome definition re-visited: old concepts and new challenges. Microbiome. 2020;8(1):103. https://doi.org/10.1186/s40168-020-00875-0.

4 Reyes A, Blanton LV, Cao S, Zhao G, Manary M, Trehan I, et al. Gut DNA viromes of Malawian twins discordant for severe acute malnutrition. Proc Natl Acad Sci U S A 2015;112(38):11941–6. https://doi.org/10.1073/pnas.1514285112.

5 Wardman JF, Bains RK, Rahfeld P, Withers SG. Carbohydrate-active enzymes (CAZymes) in the gut microbiome. Nat Rev Microbiol. 2022;20(9):542–56. https://doi.org/10.1038/s41579-022-00712-1.

6 Smith MI, Yatsunenko T, Manary MJ, Trehan I, Mkakosya R, Cheng J, et al. Gut microbiomes of Malawian twin pairs discordant for kwashiorkor. Science. 2013;339(6119):548–54. https://doi.org/10.1126/science.1229000.

7 Turnbaugh PJ, Ley RE, Mahowald MA, Magrini V, Mardis ER, Gordon JI. An obesity-associated gut microbiome with increased capacity for energy harvest. Nature. 2006;444(7122):1027–31. https://doi.org/10.1038/nature05414.

8 van Nood E, Vrieze A, Nieuwdorp M, Fuentes S, Zoetendal EG, de Vos WM, et al. Duodenal infusion of donor feces for recurrent Clostridium difficile. N Engl J Med. 2013;368(5):407–15. https://doi.org/10.1056/NEJMoa1205037.

9 Feuerstadt P, Louie TJ, Lashner B, Wang EEL, Diao L, Bryant JA, et al. SER-109, an oral microbiome therapy for recurrent *Clostridioides difficile* infection. N Engl J Med. 2022;386(3):220–9. https://doi.org/10.1056/NEJMoa2106516.

10 Donald K, Finlay BB. Early-life interactions between the microbiota and immune system: impact on immune system development and atopic disease. Nat Rev Immunol. 2023;23(11):735–48. https://doi.org/10.1038/s41577-023-00874-w.

11 van der Hee B, Wells JM. Microbial regulation of host physiology by short-chain fatty acids. Trends Microbiol. 2021;29(8):700–12. https://doi.org/10.1016/j.tim.2021.02.001.

12 Stuivenberg GA, Burton JP, Bron PA, Reid G. Why are bifidobacteria important for infants? Microorganisms. 2022;10(2):278. https://doi.org/10.3390/microorganisms10020278.

13 Dogra SK, Dore J, Damak S. Gut microbiota resilience: definition, link to health and strategies for intervention. Front Microbiol. 2020;11:572921. https://doi.org/10.3389/fmicb.2020.572921.

14 Dogra SK, Kwong Chung C, Wang D, Sakwinska O, Colombo Mottaz S, Sprenger N. Nurturing the early life gut microbiome and immune maturation for long term health. Microorganisms. 2021;9(10):2110. https://doi.org/10.3390/microorganisms9102110.

15 Stewart CJ, Ajami NJ, O'Brien JL, Hutchinson DS, Smith DP, Wong MC, et al. Temporal development of the gut microbiome in early childhood from the TEDDY study. Nature. 2018;562(7728):583–8. https://doi.org/10.1038/s41586-018-0617-x.

16 Bokulich NA, Chung J, Battaglia T, Henderson N, Jay M, Li H, et al. Antibiotics, birth mode, and diet shape microbiome maturation during early life. Sci Transl Med. 2016;8(343):343ra82. https://doi.org/10.1126/scitranslmed.aad7121.

17 Gao Y, Stokholm J, O'Hely M, Ponsonby AL, Tang MLK, Ranganathan S, et al. Gut microbiota maturity mediates the protective effect of siblings on food allergy. J Allergy Clin Immunol. 2023;152(3):667–75. https://doi.org/10.1016/j.jaci.2023.02.034.

18 Laursen MF, Zachariassen G, Bahl MI, Bergstrom A, Host A, Michaelsen KF, et al. Having older siblings is associated with gut microbiota development during early childhood. BMC Microbiol. 2015;15:154. https://doi.org/10.1186/s12866-015-0477-6.

19 Tun HM, Konya T, Takaro TK, Brook JR, Chari R, Field CJ, et al. Exposure to household furry pets influences the gut microbiota of infant at 3-4 months following various birth scenarios. Microbiome. 2017;5(1):40. https://doi.org/10.1186/s40168-017-0254-x.

20 Yatsunenko T, Rey FE, Manary MJ, Trehan I, Dominguez-Bello MG, Contreras M, et al. Human gut microbiome viewed across age and geography. Nature. 2012;486(7402):222–7. https://doi.org/10.1038/nature11053.

21 Ouyang R, Ding J, Huang Y, Zheng F, Zheng S, Ye Y, et al. Maturation of the gut metabolome during the first year of life in humans. Gut Microb. 2023;15(1):2231596. https://doi.org/10.1080/19490976.2023.2231596.

22 Xu J, Lawley B, Wong G, Otal A, Chen L, Ying TJ, et al. Ethnic diversity in infant gut microbiota is apparent before the introduction of complementary diets. Gut Microb. 2020;11(5):1362–73. https://doi.org/10.1080/19490976.2020.1756150.

23 Quin C, Gibson DL. Human behavior, not race or geography, is the strongest predictor of microbial succession in the gut bacteriome of infants. Gut Microb. 2020;11(5):1143–71. https://doi.org/10.1080/19490976.2020.1736973.

24 Stokholm J, Thorsen J, Blaser MJ, Rasmussen MA, Hjelmso M, Shah S, et al. Delivery mode and gut microbial changes correlate with an increased risk of childhood asthma. Sci Transl Med. 2020;12(569):eaax9929. https://doi.org/10.1126/scitranslmed.aax9929.

25 Galazzo G, van Best N, Bervoets L, Dapaah IO, Savelkoul PH, Hornef MW, et al. Development of the microbiota and associations with birth mode,

diet, and atopic disorders in a longitudinal analysis of stool samples, collected from infancy through early childhood. Gastroenterology. 2020;158(6): 1584–96. https://doi.org/10.1053/j.gastro.2020.01.024.

26 Bosheva M, Tokodi I, Krasnow A, Pedersen HK, Lukjancenko O, Eklund AC, et al. Infant formula with a specific blend of five human milk oligosaccharides drives the gut microbiota development and improves gut maturation markers: a randomized controlled trial. Front Nutr. 2022;9:920362. https://doi.org/10.3389/fnut.2022.920362.

27 Vatanen T, Ang QY, Siegwald L, Sarker SA, Le Roy CI, Duboux S, et al. A distinct clade of Bifidobacterium longum in the gut of Bangladeshi children thrives during weaning. Cell. 2022; 185(23):4280–97.e12. https://doi.org/10.1016/j.cell.2022.10.011.

28 Hoskinson C, Dai DLY, Del Bel KL, Becker AB, Moraes TJ, Mandhane PJ, et al. Delayed gut microbiota maturation in the first year of life is a hallmark of pediatric allergic disease. Nat Commun. 2023;14(1):4785. https://doi.org/10.1038/s41467-023-40336-4.

29 Depner M, Taft DH, Kirjavainen PV, Kalanetra KM, Karvonen AM, Peschel S, et al. Maturation of the gut microbiome during the first year of life contributes to the protective farm effect on childhood asthma. Nat Med. 2020;26(11):1766–75. https://doi.org/10.1038/s41591-020-1095-x.

30 Kostic AD, Gevers D, Siljander H, Vatanen T, Hyotylainen T, Hamalainen AM, et al. The dynamics of the human infant gut microbiome in development and in progression toward type 1 diabetes. Cell Host Microbe. 2015;17(2):260–73. https://doi.org/10.1016/j.chom.2015.01.001.

31 Dogra SK, Martin FP, Donnicola D, Julita M, Berger B, Sprenger N. Human milk oligosaccharide-stimulated *Bifidobacterium* species contribute to prevent later respiratory tract infections. Microorganisms. 2021;9(9):1939. https://doi.org/10.3390/microorganisms9091939.

32 Subramanian S, Huq S, Yatsunenko T, Haque R, Mahfuz M, Alam MA, et al. Persistent gut microbiota immaturity in malnourished Bangladeshi children. Nature. 2014;510(7505):417–21. https://doi.org/10.1038/nature13421.

33 Wan Y, Zuo T, Xu Z, Zhang F, Zhan H, Chan D, et al. Underdevelopment of the gut microbiota and bacteria species as non-invasive markers of prediction in children with autism spectrum disorder. Gut. 2022;71(5):910–8. https://doi.org/10.1136/gutjnl-2020-324015.

34 Dogra S, Sakwinska O, Soh SE, Ngom-Bru C, Bruck WM, Berger B, et al. Dynamics of infant gut microbiota are influenced by delivery mode and gestational duration and are associated with subsequent adiposity. mBio. 2015;6(1):e02419-14. https://doi.org/10.1128/mBio.02419-14.

35 Berger B, Porta N, Foata F, Grathwohl D, Delley M, Moine D, et al. Linking human milk oligosaccharides, infant fecal community types, and later risk to require antibiotics. mBio. 2020; 11(2):e03196-19. https://doi.org/10.1128/mBio.03196-19.

36 Raman AS, Gehrig JL, Venkatesh S, Chang HW, Hibberd MC, Subramanian S, et al. A sparse covarying unit that describes healthy and impaired human gut microbiota development. Science 2019; 365(6449):eaau4735. https://doi.org/10.1126/science.aau4735.

37 Ta LDH, Chan JCY, Yap GC, Purbojati RW, Drautz-Moses DI, Koh YM, et al. A compromised developmental trajectory of the infant gut microbiome and metabolome in atopic eczema. Gut Microb. 2020;12(1):1–22. https://doi.org/10.1080/19490976.2020.1801964.

38 Martin FP, Tytgat HLP, Krogh Pedersen H, Moine D, Eklund AC, Berger B, et al. Host-microbial co-metabolites modulated by human milk oligosaccharides relate to reduced risk of respiratory tract infections. Front Nutr. 2022;9:935711. https://doi.org/10.3389/fnut.2022.935711.

39 Cho S, Samuel TM, Li T, Howell BR, Baluyot K, Hazlett HC, et al. Interactions between *Bifidobacterium* and *Bacteroides* and human milk oligosaccharides and their associations with infant cognition. Front Nutr. 2023;10:1216327. https://doi.org/10.3389/fnut.2023.1216327.

Norbert Sprenger
Department of Gastrointestinal Health
Nestlé Institute of Health Sciences, Nestlé Research
Route du Jorat 57
CH-1000 Lausanne 26, Switzerland
norbert.sprenger@rdls.nestle.com

Published online: November 15, 2024

Szajewska H, Neu J, Shamir R, Wong G, Prentice AM (eds): Shaping the Future with Nutrition. Nestle Nutr Inst Workshop Ser. Basel, Karger, 2024, vol 100, pp 150–158 (DOI: 10.1159/000540146)

Integrating Next-Generation Evidence-Based Medicine Into Clinical Studies on Gut Microbiota Modulation

Hania Szajewska

Department of Paediatrics, Medical University of Warsaw, Warsaw, Poland

Abstract

This article explores the challenges and opportunities of applying Evidence-Based Medicine (EBM) to the field of gut microbiota research. EBM has revolutionized healthcare by integrating the best available evidence with clinical expertise and patient values. However, EBM has also faced criticisms such as overemphasizing results of randomized controlled trials and a lack of patient involvement. The article discusses these criticisms in the broader context of EBM and how they are particularly relevant to studies on gut health. This article also discusses the emergence of next-generation EBM methods, examining their potential strengths and limitations. For example, integrating next-generation EBM methods into gut microbiota studies offers the potential for improved understanding and patient-centered interventions. Still, it also raises questions about data quality, privacy, and patient involvement. This article concludes that as EBM evolves, careful attention must be paid to ensure that new methods are robust, transparent, and patient-centric, thereby contributing to better outcomes in gut microbiota research.

Introduction

The human gut microbiota comprises a diverse community of microorganisms, including bacteria, archaea, eukaryotes, and viruses, all residing within the gastrointestinal tract. Its role in human health is increasingly being recognized, attracting considerable attention from the scientific community and the media. In addition to the influence of diet, a range of strategies has emerged to optimize health through gut microbiota modulation, including the use of probiotics [1], prebiotics [2], synbiotics [3], postbiotics [4], and fecal microbiota transplants [5].

Evidence-based medicine (EBM) is an approach to medical practice that integrates the best available evidence with clinical expertise and patient values to make informed decisions about patient care [6]. In the context of gut microbiota research, in line with this approach, there has been a surge in randomized controlled trials (RCTs) exploring gut microbiome modifications. These trials have contributed to systematic reviews [7–9] and have shaped clinical practice guidelines [10–12]. However, the expected health benefits from these interventions are not always clear or consistent. Table 1 outlines some key challenges currently faced by clinical studies on gut microbiota modulation strategies. These challenges range from intervention specificity, where different probiotic strains produce varying outcomes, to study heterogeneity, which results in inconsistent findings due to differing study designs. Population differences, such as subjects with differing diets and existing gut microbiota composition, also complicate the generalization of results. Other issues include the short duration of many studies, difficulties in estimating appropriate sample sizes and endpoints, and the placebo effect. Further challenges include variable product quality (active ingredients or dosages) and/or viability, the lack of standardization of outcome measures across studies, and publication bias favoring positive outcomes. Some studies also lack mechanistic insights into how biotics affect conditions. At the same time, the influence of varying external factors such as diet or existing microbiota may result in interaction effects and safety concerns for specific populations such as immunocompromised children add additional layers of complexity.

This paper aims to briefly outline criticisms of EBM and address its evolving landscape, a shift accelerated by the COVID-19 pandemic. While it is discussed in the context of gut microbiota studies, the implications extend to the broader field of EBM.

Criticism of EBM

Only 15 years after the term was coined, the British Medical Journal in 2007 recognized EBM as one of the most significant medical milestones over the past 160 years, alongside breakthroughs like anesthesia, antibiotics, the discovery of

Table 1. Key challenges in clinical gut microbiota modulation pediatric research

Challenge	Examples in biotics
Intervention specificity	Different probiotic strains may have varying effects on infant colic, making it difficult to generalize findings
Study heterogeneity	Some studies on probiotics for neonatal necrotizing enterocolitis use high dosages for short durations, while others use low dosages over extended periods, leading to inconsistent results
Population differences	A synbiotic effective in European infants with gastroenteritis may not work as well in Asian infants due to differences in diet and gut microbiota composition
Short study duration	Studies showing positive effects of probiotics in reducing pediatric antibiotic-associated diarrhea after 2 weeks may not reflect long-term benefits or risks of continuous use
Power, sample size, and endpoints	Estimating appropriate sample size and power in studies involving biotics for pediatric gut health is challenging, especially for time-to-event endpoints such as time-to-relapse in conditions such as pediatric inflammatory bowel disease. Incorrect assumptions about event rates can affect the timing and interpretation of analyses
Placebo effect	Parents might report improvements in their child's gut health due to their belief in the treatment's efficacy, making it hard to attribute benefits solely to the active biotic
Variable product quality	Different brands of probiotics may contain varying active ingredients or doses, complicating comparisons in studies on pediatric constipation
Storage and viability	Probiotics that require refrigeration may lose their effectiveness if not properly stored, impacting study results
Lack of standardization	Trials assessing probiotics for pediatric irritable bowel syndrome may use different outcome measures, making comparisons difficult
Publication bias	Studies showing that synbiotics significantly reduce pediatric infectious diarrhea are more likely to be published than those with negative or inconclusive findings
Lack of mechanistic insights	A study may find that a postbiotic reduces neonatal sepsis, but not explain the underlying mechanism, making replication or application difficult
Interaction effects	The efficacy of a probiotic in preventing pediatric allergic diseases may be influenced by the child's diet or existing gut microbiota, complicating result interpretation
Safety concerns	Probiotics that benefit healthy children may cause adverse effects in immunocompromised children, raising safety concerns

DNA structure, contraception, sanitation, and vaccines [13]. Nevertheless, since its inception, EBM has not been without criticism. Below are some commonly voiced critiques of EBM [14–16]:

- **Overemphasis on results of RCTs.** Critics argue that EBM places too much emphasis on RCTs as the gold standard of evidence, potentially ignoring valuable insights from other research designs such as observational studies or expert clinical judgment.
- **Devaluation of clinical experience.** EBMs emphasis on empirical research data can lead one to undervalue the importance of clinical experience and individualized patient care.
- **Limited applicability.** Clinical studies often focus on narrowly defined populations, and their findings may not be directly applicable to patients with multiple comorbidities or those who are outside the study's demographic scope.

- **Bias and conflict of interest.** Some studies included in EBM reviews might be funded by pharmaceutical companies or other entities with vested interests, potentially leading to bias in study design, interpretation, or reporting.
- **Overdiagnosis and overtreatment.** EBM can sometimes contribute to a culture of overdiagnosis and overtreatment, particularly when guidelines recommend interventions for conditions that might not require them.
- **Time consuming.** Keeping up with the latest evidence can be time-consuming for healthcare practitioners under significant time constraints.
- **Rigidity.** Critics argue that EBM can be overly rigid and reductionist, focusing on specific interventions for specific conditions rather than considering the holistic context of patient care.
- **Access to evidence.** Not all healthcare practitioners have access to the latest research articles and systematic reviews, making it challenging to practice EBM in some settings.
- **Lack of patient voice.** Some critics argue that EBM does not adequately consider patient preferences, values, and unique circumstances.
- **Dependence on quality research.** The quality of EBM is dependent on the quality of the underlying research, which may have limitations such as small sample sizes, short follow-up periods, or inadequate controls.

The Evolution of EBM: A New Generation Emerges

Recognizing the Need for Change

The existing critiques of EBM have served as catalysts for its evolution. Although calls for reform were already in place, the COVID-19 pandemic further intensified the urgency for change [17, 18].

Historical Criticism and Proposed Solutions

In 2014, Trisha Greenhalgh and colleagues [19] identified major issues with EBM: the outsized influence of pharmaceutical companies on research, the overwhelming amount of available evidence, a focus on minor treatment differences in studies, physicians' rigid adherence to algorithms, and the inadequacy of a one-size-fits-all approach for diverse patient populations. To tackle these challenges, the authors advocated for more personalized patient care integrating evidence and values, more clinically relevant research, and reducing the impact of commercial interests.

The EBM Manifesto

A significant effort to improve EBM was the EBM manifesto, jointly published by *The BMJ* [20] and the University of Oxford's Centre for Evidence-Based Medicine. The manifesto calls for a response to systematic bias, wastage, error, and fraud in research underpinning patient care. It provides a guide to improve the quality of evidence by tackling challenges such as poorly conducted studies, incomplete or selective release of research findings, and conflicts of interest from commercial and academic sectors.

The Role of COVID-19

The COVID-19 crisis underscored the urgency for quick decisions in an ever-changing global landscape. A recent article in *BMJ Evidence-Based Medicine* [21] examined the shortcomings of conventional EBM in the face of such dynamic and complex scenarios. The authors suggest broadening the criteria and expanding the definition for what is considered "high-quality" evidence and propose incorporating methodologies from diverse fields such as complexity science and engineering under the umbrella of mechanistic research. They argue that these new approaches, colloquially known as "EBM+," could synergize with existing EBM methods to create the multidisciplinary evidence base needed for effectively navigating ongoing and future challenges.

Next-Generation EBM

A recent article in *Nature Medicine* [22], entitled "The Next Generation of Evidence-Based Medicine," explores how emerging technologies and methodologies could revolutionize medical practice. The paper emphasizes the transformative potential of wearable technologies, data science, and machine learning to create a more holistic and personalized form of evidence-based medicine. While acknowledging that the COVID-19 pandemic revealed existing limitations in the traditional clinical trial model, the authors point out that it also catalyzed positive shifts. These include the development of innovative trial designs and transitioning toward a more patient-focused and intuitive system for generating evidence.

Next-Generation EBM in the Context of Gut Microbiota Studies

In the evolving landscape of EBM, various innovative methods have the potential to significantly impact research in the field of gut microbiota and biotics. Real-World Data and Real-World Evidence [23] could be employed for observational studies to examine the long-term health effects of consumption of biotics, using data sources such as electronic health records. Similarly, the digitalization of clinical trials [24] offers the possibility of more patient-centered monitoring through the use of wearable devices [25] to track symptoms such as bowel movements, bloating, or colic. The development and use of agreed-upon Core Outcome Sets present the opportunity for standardizing measurements across trials, aiding in the comparability of studies [26]. Patient-Centered Outcomes [27] could be developed and used to reflect the metrics most relevant to patients, such as gastrointestinal comfort or quality of life. Adaptive Trial Designs [28] have the potential to bring flexibility to research, allowing study protocols to be adjusted based on interim results. This could be especially beneficial for fine-tuning biotics' dosages in conditions such as inflammatory bowel disease. The use of Master Protocols [29] could streamline multiple sub-studies under a single plan, improving coordination and resource allocation. Pragmatic Trials [30] offer a pathway for assessing the real-world applicability of biotics in clinical settings. The application of Artificial Intelligence (AI) and Machine Learning techniques [31] to clinical trials could be utilized for complex

Table 2. Methods in next-generation EBM with examples in the field of biotics

Method	Description	Potential use in the field of biotics
Real-World Data/ Real-World Evidence (RWD/RWE)	RWD: Data collected from sources such as electronic health records, billing data, registries, and patient-generated data that inform health status RWE: Clinical evidence from RWD analysis about a medical product's use, benefits, or risks, sourced from various study designs or analyses	Observational studies analyzing the health effects of long-term consumption of biotics using data from electronic health records
Digitalization of Clinical Trials	Use of digital tools to enhance the efficiency and patient-centeredness of clinical trials	Clinical trials using wearable devices to monitor bowel movement and bloating in patients taking biotics or fecal microbiota transplants
Core Outcome Sets (COS)	Agreed-upon sets of outcomes that should be measured and reported in all clinical trials for a specific condition	Adoption of COS for measuring outcomes in trials assessing the effects of biotics on irritable bowel syndrome
Patient-Centered Outcomes	Focus on outcomes that matter most to patients	Studies evaluating patient's gastrointestinal comfort or quality of life after intake of biotics
Adaptive Trial Designs	Clinical trials that allow modifications to the procedures based on interim results	Adaptive trials testing different doses of biotics in patients with inflammatory bowel disease
Master Protocols	Master protocols are single plans for multiple sub-studies, such as Basket, Umbrella, and Platform Trials, that save resources and improve coordination compared to separate trials	Platform trials testing multiple probiotics against a common control group in patients with irritable bowel syndrome
Pragmatic Trials	Clinical trials designed to test the effectiveness of interventions in real-world clinical practice settings	Pragmatic trials assessing the real-world effectiveness of biotics in patients with functional dyspepsia
Artificial Intelligence and Machine Learning	Use of advanced computational techniques to analyze complex data sets and predict outcomes	Machine learning models predicting the efficacy of specific biotics in altering gut microbiota composition
Social Media and Online Community Research	Utilization of social media platforms and online communities to increase awareness of clinical trials and engage underrepresented populations	Promoting biotics clinical trials for pediatric gastrointestinal issues on social media such as X (formerly Twitter) and Facebook to reach rural parents. Engaging adolescents in online communities for gut health studies

data analysis, providing predictive insights into how specific biotics might influence gut microbiota composition. Finally, various forms of social media are emerging as potential tools for boosting awareness and engagement in clinical trials, particularly among underrepresented populations including rural parents and adolescents. Table 2 presents a detailed overview of these next-generation EBM methods and their potential applications in the specialized field of biotics and gut microbiota research.

Challenges of Next-Generation EBM

The next-generation EBM holds great promise. However, there are many unknowns. For example, the incorporation of big data, including Real-World Data/Real-World Evidence and data from electronic health records, wearables, and social media, raises questions about data quality, privacy, and the appropriate statistical methods for analyzing these large, heterogeneous datasets. The potential of AI to revolutionize EBM is significant, but there are uncertainties about the transparency, interpretability, and reliability of AI-driven analyses and recommendations. While patient involvement in decision-making is a core principle of EBM, the practicalities of how best to involve patients (or their care providers in the case of infants and young children), consider their preferences, and integrate their insights into the evidence base are still being explored.

Conclusions

Incorporating next-generation EBM methodologies in gut microbiota studies offers exciting avenues for both understanding and delivering more patient-oriented treatments. While these innovative methods address some limitations of traditional EBM, such as rigid study designs and limited patient involvement, they bring along their own set of challenges. These include issues related to data quality, privacy concerns, and the complexities of effective patient engagement, especially when utilizing new data sources such as wearables and social media. As EBM continues to evolve, it becomes crucial to address these challenges head-on, ensuring that the methodologies employed are not only robust and evidence-driven but also transparent and responsive to patient needs. Future research should aim to develop strategies to mitigate these challenges, ensuring that EBM remains a powerful tool for improving gut health outcomes for diverse patient populations.

Conflict of Interest Statement

This article represents a summary of a presentation made by the author at the 100th Nestlé Nutrition Institute Workshop, for which an honorarium was paid.

References

1 Hill C, Guarner F, Reid G, Gibson GR, Merenstein DJ, Pot B, et al. Expert consensus document. The International Scientific Association for Probiotics and Prebiotics consensus statement on the scope and appropriate use of the term probiotic. Nat Rev Gastroenterol Hepatol. 2014;11(8):506–14. https://doi.org/10.1038/nrgastro.2014.66.

2 Gibson GR, Hutkins R, Sanders ME, Prescott SL, Reimer RA, Salminen SJ, et al. Expert consensus document: the International Scientific Association for Probiotics and Prebiotics (ISAPP) consensus statement on the definition and scope of prebiotics. Nat Rev Gastroenterol Hepatol. 2017;14(8):491–502. https://doi.org/10.1038/nrgastro.2017.75.

3 Swanson KS, Gibson GR, Hutkins R, Reimer RA, Reid G, Verbeke K, et al. The International Scientific Association for Probiotics and Prebiotics (ISAPP) consensus statement on the definition and scope of synbiotics. Nat Rev Gastroenterol Hepatol. 2020;17(11):687–701. https://doi.org/10.1038/s41575-020-0344-2.

4 Salminen S, Collado MC, Endo A, Hill C, Lebeer S, Quigley EMM, et al. The International Scientific Association of Probiotics and Prebiotics (ISAPP) consensus statement on the definition and scope of postbiotics. Nat Rev Gastroenterol Hepatol. 2021;18(9):649–67. https://doi.org/10.1038/s41575-021-00440-6.

5 Krajicek E, Fischer M, Allegretti JR, Kelly CR. Nuts and bolts of fecal microbiota transplantation. Clin Gastroenterol Hepatol. 2019;17(2):345–52. https://doi.org/10.1016/j.cgh.2018.09.029.

6 Sackett DL, Rosenberg WM, Gray JA, Haynes RB, Richardson WS. Evidence based medicine: what it is and what it isn't. BMJ. 1996;312(7023):71–2. https://doi.org/10.1136/bmj.312.7023.71.

7 Collinson S, Deans A, Padua-Zamora A, Gregorio GV, Li C, Dans LF, et al. Probiotics for treating acute infectious diarrhoea. Cochrane Database Syst Rev. 2020;12:CD003048. https://doi.org/10.1002/14651858.CD003048.pub4.

8 Sharif S, Meader N, Oddie SJ, Rojas-Reyes MX, McGuire W. Probiotics to prevent necrotising enterocolitis in very preterm or very low birth weight infants. Cochrane Database Syst Rev. 2023;7:CD005496. https://doi.org/10.1002/14651858.CD005496.pub6.

9 Guo Q, Goldenberg JZ, Humphrey C, El Dib R, Johnston BC. Probiotics for the prevention of pediatric antibiotic-associated diarrhea. Cochrane Database Syst Rev. 2019;4:CD004827. https://doi.org/10.1002/14651858.CD004827.pub5.

10 Szajewska H, Berni Canani R, Domellöf M, Guarino A, Hojsak I, Indrio F, et al. Probiotics for the management of pediatric gastrointestinal disorders: position paper of the ESPGHAN special interest group on gut microbiota and modifications. J Pediatr Gastroenterol Nutr. 2023;76(2):232–47. https://doi.org/10.1097/MPG.0000000000003633.

11 Su GL, Ko CW, Bercik P, Falck-Ytter Y, Sultan S, Weizman AV, et al. AGA clinical practice guidelines on the role of probiotics in the management of gastrointestinal disorders. Gastroenterology. 2020;159(2):697–705. https://doi.org/10.1053/j.gastro.2020.05.059.

12 Hojsak I, Kolaček S, Mihatsch W, Mosca A, Shamir R, Szajewska H, et al. Synbiotics in the management of pediatric gastrointestinal disorders: position paper of the ESPGHAN special interest group on gut microbiota and modifications. J Pediatr Gastroenterol Nutr. 2023;76(1):102–8. https://doi.org/10.1097/MPG.0000000000003568.

13 Dickersin K, Straus SE, Bero LA. Evidence based medicine: increasing, not dictating, choice. BMJ. 2007;334(suppl 1):s10. https://doi.org/10.1136/bmj.39062.639444.94.

14 Ratnani I, Fatima S, Abid MM, Surani Z, Surani S. Evidence-based medicine: history, review, criticisms, and pitfalls. Cureus. 2023;15(2):e35266. https://doi.org/10.7759/cureus.35266.

15 Hannes K, Aertgeerts B, Schepers R, Goedhuys J, Buntinx F. Evidence-based medicine: a discussion of the most frequently occurring criticisms. Ned Tijdschr Geneeskd. 2005;149(36):1983–8.

16 Cohen AM, Stavri PZ, Hersh WR. A categorization and analysis of the criticisms of evidence-based medicine. Int J Med Inform. 2004;73(1):35–43. https://doi.org/10.1016/j.ijmedinf.2003.11.002.

17 Pearson H. How COVID broke the evidence pipeline. Nature. 2021;593(7858):182–5. https://doi.org/10.1038/d41586-021-01246-x.

18 Gaba P, Bhatt DL. The COVID-19 pandemic: a catalyst to improve clinical trials. Nat Rev Cardiol. 2020;17(11):673–5. https://doi.org/10.1038/s41569-020-00439-7.

19 Greenhalgh T, Howick J, Maskrey N, Evidence Based Medicine Renaissance Group. Evidence based medicine: a movement in crisis? BMJ. 2014; 348:g3725. https://doi.org/10.1136/bmj.g3725.

20 Heneghan C, Mahtani KR, Goldacre B, Godlee F, Macdonald H, Jarvies D. Evidence based medicine manifesto for better healthcare. BMJ. 2017;357: j2973. https://doi.org/10.1136/bmj.j2973.

21 Greenhalgh T, Fisman D, Cane DJ, Oliver M, Macintyre CR. Adapt or die: how the pandemic made the shift from EBM to EBM+ more urgent. BMJ Evid Based Med. 2022;27(5):253–60. https://doi.org/10.1136/bmjebm-2022-111952.

22 Subbiah V. The next generation of evidence-based medicine. Nat Med. 2023;29(1):49–58. https://doi.org/10.1038/s41591-022-02160-z.

23 FDA. Real-World Evidence. 2023.

24 Inan OT, Tenaerts P, Prindiville SA, Reynolds HR, Dizon DS, Cooper-Arnold K, et al. Digitizing clinical trials. NPJ Digit Med. 2020;3:101. https://doi.org/10.1038/s41746-020-0302-y.

25 Smuck M, Odonkor CA, Wilt JK, Schmidt N, Swiernik MA. The emerging clinical role of wearables: factors for successful implementation in healthcare. NPJ Digit Med. 2021;4(1):45. https://doi.org/10.1038/s41746-021-00418-3.

26 Kirkham JJ, Williamson P. Core outcome sets in medical research. BMJ Med. 2022;1: e000284. https://doi.org/10.1136/bmjmed-2022-000284.

27 Tringale M, Stephen G, Boylan AM, Heneghan C. Integrating patient values and preferences in healthcare: a systematic review of qualitative evidence. BMJ Open. 2022;12(11): e067268. https://doi.org/10.1136/bmjopen-2022-067268.

28 Bhatt DL, Mehta C. Adaptive designs for clinical trials. N Engl J Med. 2016;375(1):65–74. https://doi.org/10.1056/NEJMra1510061.

29 Woodcock J, LaVange LM. Master protocols to study multiple therapies, multiple diseases, or both. N Engl J Med. 2017;377(1):62–70. https://doi.org/10.1056/NEJMra1510062.

30 Ford I, Norrie J. Pragmatic trials. N Engl J Med. 2016;375(5):454–63. https://doi.org/10.1056/NEJMra1510059.

31 Askin S, Burkhalter D, Calado G, El Dakrouni S. Artificial Intelligence Applied to clinical trials: opportunities and challenges. Health Technol (Berl). 2023;13(2):203–13. https://doi.org/10.1007/s12553-023-00738-2.

Hania Szajewska
Department of Paediatrics, Medical University of Warsaw
Żwirki i Wigury 63A, 02-091 Warsaw, Poland
hszajewska@wum.edu.pl

Published online: November 15, 2024

Szajewska H, Neu J, Shamir R, Wong G, Prentice AM (eds): Shaping the Future with Nutrition. Nestle Nutr Inst Workshop Ser. Basel, Karger, 2024, vol 100, pp 159–169 (DOI: 10.1159/000540147)

Nutrition Challenges and Opportunities When Shifting to Plant-Based Diets

Paula Hallam

Plant Based Kids Ltd., Kingston upon Thames, UK

Abstract

There has been a significant increase in the number of people shifting towards plant-based dietary patterns over the past decade due to interest in protecting the health of the planet as well as improving human health. Studies have shown that vegetarian diets are associated with a lower prevalence of obesity in adults and children; therefore, moving towards a vegetarian diet in childhood may help prevent obesity later in life. The VeChi study in Germany found that on average vegetarian and vegan children grew equally well as omnivorous children. It is important to ensure that children following plant-based diets have adequate amounts of key nutrients, such as energy, fats, iron, calcium, iodine, vitamin B12, and omega-3 fats. In the VeChi studies, vegan children had the lowest intakes of calcium and iodine out of the three diet groups. The vegan children also had the lowest vitamin B12 intakes without supplements, but when supplements were taken into account, they had the highest vitamin B12 intakes. Iron intake in vegetarian children is consistently reported as higher than in omnivorous children. However, iron stores (indicated by low ferritin levels) tend to be lower in vegetarian compared to omnivorous children, due to decreased bioavailability of non-haem iron found in plant foods. When introducing solids, iron-rich foods should be offered early and paired with iron enhancers such as vitamin C and beta-carotene to improve iron absorption.

Introduction

Plant-based eating patterns have become increasingly popular around the world, particularly over the past decade. In the UK, The Vegan Society reported that the number of people following a vegan diet quadrupled from 2014 to 2019. Additionally, a more recent survey by The Vegan Society in May 2021 revealed that 1 in 4 British people had reduced the amount of animal products they were consuming since the start of the COVID-19 pandemic [1]. The sign-ups for the Veganuary campaign – where people eat vegan for the month of January – hit record highs in 2023, with over 700,000 people signing up from almost every country in the world, compared to 3,000 participants in 2014, the year the Veganuary campaign started [2].

These statistics illustrate that there are huge numbers of people who are interested in trying out a vegan lifestyle, and many are sticking with it: according to the 2022 Veganuary statistics, 83% of participants who were not already vegan said they would be permanently changing their diet, either by becoming vegan or halving the amount of animal products they eat [2].

Plant-Based Eating Patterns and Children

The nutritional requirements of infants and children are different from adults, as they are growing and developing rapidly. Therefore, their nutritional requirements need to be carefully considered and meals planned accordingly. Both the British Dietetic Association and the Academy of Nutrition and Dietetics in the United States have produced statements in support of the safety of vegan and vegetarian diets for children:

> "It is the position of the Academy of Nutrition and Dietetics that appropriately planned vegetarian diets, including total vegetarian or vegan diets, are healthful, nutritionally adequate, and may provide health benefits in the prevention and treatment of certain diseases. Well-planned vegetarian diets are appropriate for individuals during all stages of the lifecycle, including pregnancy, lactation, infancy, childhood, adolescence, and for athletes" [3].

> "A balanced vegan diet can be enjoyed by children and adults, including during pregnancy and breastfeeding, if the nutritional intake is well-planned" [4].

What Does "Plant-Based" Actually Mean?

There is no one universally agreed definition for "plant-based", however, the British Nutrition Foundation defines a plant-based eating pattern as an eating pattern that has *"a greater emphasis on foods derived from plants, such as fruits and vegetables, wholegrains, pulses, nuts, seeds, and oils"* [5]. Plant-based diets are not the same as vegetarian or vegan diets and they do not necessarily mean only plants but rather proportionately more foods are chosen from plant sources [6] (Table 1).

Nutrition Opportunities

Increased Micronutrient Intake

Plant-based diets are often criticized for lacking certain micronutrients but they are actually abundant in many vitamins and minerals. The VeChi study [7] found that the vegan children had the highest intakes of beta-carotene, vitamins E, C, B1, B6, folate, potassium, magnesium, and iron, with vegetarian children having the next highest intakes and omnivorous children having the lowest intakes of these micronutrients.

Almost one-third (29%) of children in the UK aged 5 to 10 years eat less than one portion of vegetables per day, with those living in the poorest conditions eating the fewest vegetables [8]. Less than 1 in 5 (18%) of children aged 5 to 15 years eat 5 portions of fruit and vegetables per day in England, according to the Health Survey for England [9]. Encouraging children to include more plant-based foods in their eating patterns could increase their micronutrient intake and subsequently improve their health outcomes.

Table 1. Definitions of different types of plant-based diets [6]

Dietary pattern	Summary of foods excluded/included in the diet
Flexitarian	primarily/mostly vegetarian but may eat some meat, fish/seafood, poultry, dairy and eggs occasionally
Pescatarian	excludes meat and poultry but includes fish/seafood, dairy and eggs
Lacto-vegetarian	excludes meat, fish/seafood, poultry and eggs but includes dairy products
Ovo-vegetarian	excludes meat, fish/seafood, poultry and dairy products, but includes eggs
Lacto-ovo vegetarian	excludes meat, fish/seafood and poultry but include eggs and dairy products
Vegan	excludes all animal products including meat, fish/seafood, poultry, eggs, dairy and honey

Intakes of some other micronutrients such as calcium, iodine, vitamin B2, and vitamin B12 have been found to be lower in children following vegan, vegetarian, and predominantly plant-based diets [7]. These micronutrients and how to ensure an adequate intake for plant-based children will be discussed further in the "ensuring adequate intakes of key nutrients" section.

Decreased Risk of Overweight and Obesity

Around the world, childhood obesity is a major public health concern. In the UK national measurement program in 2021/22, 10% of children aged 4 to 5 years were obese and a further 12% were overweight. For children aged 10 to 11 years, the figures were even higher with almost 1 in 4 (23.4%) being classed as obese and a further 14.3% classed as overweight [10]. High intakes of protein (particularly dairy protein) during infancy and early childhood (10%–15% of energy intake or more) have been consistently associated with increased weight gain and a higher risk of later overweight and obesity [11]. In another study [12], the ages of 12 months and 5 to 6 years of age were identified as critical ages for later obesity development, where higher total and animal protein (but not vegetable protein) was positively associated with later body fatness. This is why it is recommended that cow's milk (and other animal milks) be limited to around 2 cups per day after 12 months of age if included in the diet.

Epidemiological studies have shown that vegetarian diets are associated with a lower body mass index (BMI) and a lower prevalence of obesity in adults and children [13]. Vegetarian children tend to be leaner than non-vegetarian children and their BMI difference becomes greater during adolescence [13]. A plant-based eating pattern in childhood could be an approach to prevent overweight and obesity later in life.

Increased Fiber Intake

Most adults in affluent societies do not consume enough fiber, with the average daily fiber intake for adults being 20 g/d [14], compared to the recommended fiber intake for adults of 30 g/d [14]. Data from the National Diet and Nutrition Survey indicate that children are also not consuming enough fiber, with 1.5 to 3 year olds average fiber intake being 10 g/d, 4 to 10 year olds 14 g/d, and 11 to 18 year olds 16 g/d. According to the Scientific Advisory Committee on Nutrition report on carbohydrates [14], recommended fiber intakes for children aged 2 to 5 years are 15 g/d, 5 to 11 years are 20 g/d and 11 to 18 years are 25 g/d.

Plant-based diets are generally higher in fiber than "standard" omnivorous diets. In the VeChi study, the vegan group of children had the highest fiber intake with an average intake of 21.9 g fiber per day, compared to 14.7 g/d in the vegetarian group and 12 g/d in the omnivorous group [15].

Although eating a sufficient amount of fiber has many health benefits for a healthy gut microbiome, this needs to be balanced with infants and young children's need for energy-dense foods in order to meet their relatively high energy requirements to support their growth and development. Fiber has a satiating effect and therefore young children could be at risk of not achieving adequate energy intakes if they fill up too quickly on high-fiber foods. Fiber recommendations are only set from 2 years of age in the UK [14] and therefore a gradual introduction and increase in fiber from introducing solids at around 6 months to 2 years of age seems sensible.

Nutrition Challenges

Children's Growth

Recent studies looking at children's growth when following vegan or vegetarian diets include the VeChi study of 1- to 3-year-olds [7] and the VeChi youth study of 6- to 18-year-olds [15], both from Germany. The VeChi study concluded that vegan and vegetarian diets provided sufficient energy and nutrients for adequate growth, similar growth to omnivorous children. There was a small percentage of vegan and vegetarian children who were classified as stunted. However, all of these cases could be explained by extended breastfeeding without the introduction of appropriate, nutrient and energy-dense complementary foods. This is why it is so important to ensure that infants and young children are offered sufficient energy-dense foods to support their growth.

In the VeChi youth study [15], which included 401 children (150 in the vegetarian group, 114 in the vegan group, and 137 in the omnivorous group) with a mean age of 12.7 ± 3.9 years (age range 5.5–19.1 years) there was no statistical difference between the diet groups in terms of their mean weights, heights, and BMI z-scores. The mean weight for the diet groups was 45 kg, 43 kg, and 46 kg for the vegetarian, vegan, and omnivorous groups respectively (*p* value 0.49). The mean height for the diet groups was 154 cm, 152 cm, and 156 cm for the vegetarian, vegan, and omnivorous groups respectively (*p* value 0.49). The mean BMI-SDS was −0.3 ± 0.9, −0.6 ± 0.9, and −0.3 ± 1.0 for the vegetarian, vegan, and omnivorous groups, respectively (*p* value 0.15).

Introducing Allergens – What about Animal-Based Allergens?

Food allergy is estimated to affect as many as 8% of children in the United States and 7% of children in Canada [16]. The prevalence of food allergies, especially peanut allergies, appears to be increasing worldwide, including in developing countries [17]. Food allergies can result in significant morbidity and psychosocial burden, so preventing food allergies should be a public health priority.

There is a growing body of evidence to suggest that introducing food allergens – particularly eggs and peanuts – to infants from around 6 months of age may help prevent allergies to those foods from developing later in life [17–19]. The "top 9" food allergens include cow's milk/dairy products, eggs, peanuts, tree nuts, wheat, soya, sesame, fish, and shellfish. Four out of these top nine foods are animal-based, which presents a dilemma for plant-based families who may not wish to introduce animal-based foods to their children for ethical reasons. When plant-based families are considering whether to introduce animal-based allergens, it may be helpful to consider the following points.

1. Food Allergy Risk Factors
There is no international consensus on the exact definition of what qualifies an infant as "high risk" of developing a food allergy [16]. In the NIAID guidelines for the prevention of peanut allergy [20], an infant was defined as "high risk" of developing peanut allergy if they had severe eczema and/or an egg allergy. Severe eczema is widely considered to be a significant risk factor for developing a food allergy [20]. It is worth mentioning that no infant is considered at "no risk" of developing a food allergy but rather "standard risk".

2. Maintenance of Allergen Intake
It is not sufficient to introduce a food allergen to an infant once, twice, or even three times only. Once a food allergen has been introduced to an infant in an age-appropriate portion, it needs to be offered regularly (at least once or twice per week) for a number of years to maintain tolerance to that allergen. It is not known exactly how long the weekly allergen exposure needs to continue. In the LEAP study [18] they maintained exposure (or avoidance) of peanut protein for 5 years and then there was a trial of 1-year peanut protein avoidance for both groups. There was not an increase in peanut allergy prevalence after this avoidance period so this would suggest that 5 years was enough time to establish immune tolerance. However, it is not known if this can be extrapolated to other allergens. In addition, the participants in the LEAP study [18] were considered at "high risk" for developing peanut allergy as they had early onset eczema and/or an egg allergy. In plant-based families who are not including any animal products, it may not be feasible to continue the exposure to an animal-based allergen.

Ensuring Adequate Intakes of Key Nutrients

In the following section, I will discuss the key nutrients for infants and young children and how to ensure adequate intake of these nutrients from plant-based sources and/or supplements. Plant-based diets tend to be rich in beta-carotene, vitamins E, C, and B1, folate, magnesium potassium, fiber, and phytochemicals, as reported by the VeChi studies [7, 15]. On the other hand, plant-based diets, particularly vegan diets, can be potentially low in critical nutrients such as energy, protein, fats, omega-3 fats, calcium, iodine, vitamin D, and vitamin B12. It is important that parents are aware of these potential shortfalls and how to plan the nutritional intake of their children including the need for supplements.

Fats

Fats are an important source of calories in infants and young children and they have a higher requirement for fat than adults, as a percentage of calorie intake. For adults and children over the age of 4 years, the recommended fat intake is "not more than 35%" of their calories [21], whereas infants and young children need proportionately more fats, around 35% to 45% of energy intake as they play an important structural role in cell membranes of all tissues and are particularly important in brain, eye and other neural tissues [22]. Many plant foods are naturally low in fats, such as beans, lentils, (most) fruits and vegetables. Therefore it is important to emphasize plant sources of fats such as avocado, nut butters or ground nuts, seed butters or ground seeds, olive oil, as well as breast milk and higher-fat dairy alternatives as important sources of fats and calories.

Omega-3 Fats

In addition, plant foods do not contain the long-chain fats docosahexaenoic acid (DHA) and eicosapentaenoic acid (EPA), only the precursor essential fatty acid alpha-linolenic acid (ALA). ALA is found in walnuts, chia, hemp, and flaxseeds and their oils. A DHA/EPA supplement derived from algal oil is recommended for breastfeeding women and children from 1 year of age as the conversion of ALA to DHA and EPA is not very efficient [22]. 100 mg DHA per day is recommended from 1 year of age and 400 to 500 mg DHA/EPA combined (with at least 250 mg being from DHA) for breastfeeding women [23, 24].

Protein

It is widely believed among both the general public and health professionals, that certain plant foods are completely missing specific amino acids and therefore protein adequacy cannot be achieved by plant foods alone. All plant foods contain all 20 amino acids including the 9 essential amino acids [25] albeit in different proportions.

As long as a reasonable variety of foods are eaten and energy requirements are met, protein requirements can easily be achieved by eating mostly or all plant foods [26]. Excellent sources of plant protein include soya foods such as soya drinks, tofu, tempeh, and edamame beans; other beans, lentils, peas, ground nuts/seeds or nut/seed butters and cereals/grains, particularly quinoa, wheat, and oats.

Iron

Iron is one of the main nutritional reasons for introducing solids to infants, as stores that they were born with start to deplete from birth so that by 6 months of age, if born at full term and with good birth weight [27], infants are at risk of iron deficiency and therefore need to be offered dietary sources of iron. Iron intakes in vegetarian children are consistently reported as higher than in omnivorous children [7, 15], however, iron stores (indicated by low ferritin levels) tend to be lower in vegetarian compared to omnivorous children, due to lower bioavailability of non-haem iron found in plant foods [28]. When introducing solids, iron-rich foods should be offered early and paired with iron enhancers such as vitamin C and beta-carotene to improve iron absorption. Examples of iron-rich foods include legumes (beans, lentils, peas, soya beans), tofu, nut butters or ground nuts, seed butters or ground seeds, dried fruits (particularly dried figs, apricots, and dates), and grains such as quinoa, oats, and iron-fortified cereals. Vitamin C-rich foods include strawberries, kiwi fruit, tomatoes, peppers, broccoli, potatoes and citrus fruits.

Calcium and Vitamin D

There have been several studies illustrating that vegan children have lower calcium intakes than vegetarian and omnivorous children [7, 15]. Desmond et al. [29] also reported lower bone mineral content in vegan children, although calcium (and vitamin D) intakes were not reported. Another study found that vegan diets were not associated with an increased fracture risk as long as calcium intake was adequate [30]. Therefore, it is important to ensure that children following plant-based diets have adequate calcium (and vitamin D) intakes to protect their bone health. Fortified dairy alternative drinks can provide concentrated and convenient sources of bioavailable calcium.

Vitamin B12

All vegan infants, children, and adults, including and especially breastfeeding women, should ensure that they have adequate vitamin B12 intakes as plant foods do not contain vitamin B12 (unless fortified). See Table 2 for supplement dosages recommended.

In the VeChi study [7] the vegan children had the lowest vitamin B12 intakes without supplements, but when supplements were taken into account, they had the highest vitamin B12 intakes.

Table 2. Summary of nutritional recommendations for plant-based children

Key nutrients to consider	Plant-based sources	Additional considerations
Iron	Beans, lentils, tofu, soya beans, iron-fortified cereals, nuts and seeds[a] (Eggs)	Pair with foods rich in vitamin C and beta-carotene to maximise iron absorption
Protein	Beans, lentils, tofu, tempeh, soya beans, nuts and seeds[a], cereals and grains, quinoa, soya/pea based dairy alternatives (Dairy products and eggs)	Aim to offer a variety of sources over 24 h
Fats	Avocados, nuts and seeds[a], plant oils e.g., Olive oil, rapeseed oil (Full fat dairy products and egg yolks)	Aim to offer at each meal to ensure adequate energy intakes
Calcium	Breast milk or infant formula[b] Fortified dairy alternative drinks and yoghurts, fortified cereals, calcium-set tofu, tahini, dried figs, almonds, low oxalate vegetables such as broccoli, kale, pak choi, spring greens	Aim to offer 2–3 calcium-rich foods per day for children 1–3 years and 3–4 per day for children 4–6 years of age
DHA/EPA	Algal oil (Oily fish if included for example in pescatarian diets)	Supplement recommended **400–500 mg DHA/EPA combined per day** (with at least 250 mg as DHA) for breastfeeding women **100 mg DHA per day** from 1 year of age
Vitamin B12	Fortified plant foods (Dairy products, eggs, fish)	Supplement recommended **2.5–5 µg/d** from around 7 months of age **10–25 µg/d** for breastfeeding women
Iodine	Iodised salt (not widely available in the UK) Seaweed - can contain excessive quantities so not recommended for children and pregnant women (Dairy products, fish and shellfish)	Supplement recommended **50–70 µg/d** from 1 year of age **150–200 µg/d** for breastfeeding women **Please note** Some plant milks are fortified with iodine and in some cases can cover iodine requirements. Please check the label

[a]No whole nuts or large seeds – use ground nuts/seeds or smooth nut/seed butters for children under 4 years.
[b]BM or infant formula are the only suitable main drinks for infants under 12 months. Dairy products or fortified alternatives can be used within foods from 6 months of age.
(Foods in brackets may be included in vegetarian or pescatarian diets).
Supplement recommendations references: [23, 24].

Iodine

Iodine intakes were found to be low in all three diet groups in the VeChi studies including the omnivorous children. A 2009 study in the UK [31] looking at the iodine status of more than 800 14- to 15-year-old girls found that there were significant numbers of girls that were iodine deficient. Urinary iodine measurements were used and they indicated that 51% of participants had mild iodine deficiency, 16% had moderate deficiency and 1% had severe deficiency. The participants were omnivorous. So low iodine intakes are not exclusively a problem in vegan/vegetarian children. The main dietary sources of iodine are cow's milk and dairy products as well as fish and shellfish with a small amount present in eggs [32]. If a child is following a vegan diet, all these sources of iodine will be excluded. Seaweed is a plant-based source of iodine but levels can vary widely with some varieties containing excessive quantities, therefore seaweed is not generally recommended as an iodine source for children. An iodine supplement is the best way to ensure an adequate (and not excessive) iodine intake.

Recommendations and Conclusions

It is possible to provide all the nutrient requirements for infants and children on plant-based diets including vegan and vegetarian diets as long as the diet is well planned and nutritional knowledge is required by parents/carers as well as selected supplements for children on vegan diets especially. For future research, it would be helpful to have longer-term studies looking at children's growth, development, and nutritional status longitudinally when infants are raised on a vegan diet from birth.

Meal planning resources such as the one produced by Menal-Puey et al. may be helpful when health professionals are counseling vegan/vegetarian families on how to provide adequate nutrition for children [33].

Conflict of Interest Statement

The author declares that she follows a vegetarian diet herself. No other conflicts of interest. The author received lecture honoraria and travel reimbursement from Nestlé Nutrition Institute.

References

1 https://www.vegansociety.com/news/media/statistics/worldwide

2 https://veganuary.com/83-of-veganuary-2022-participants-plan-permanent-diet-change/

3 Melina V, Craig W, Levin S. Position of the academy of nutrition and dietetics: vegetarian diets. J Acad Nutr Diet. 2016;116(12):1970–80. https://doi.org/10.1016/j.jand.2016.09.025.

4 https://www.bda.uk.com/resource/british-dietetic-association-confirms-well-planned-vegan-diets-can-support-healthy-living-in-people-of-all-ages.html

5 https://www.nutrition.org.uk/putting-it-into-practice/plant-based-diets/plant-based-diets/

6 https://www.bda.uk.com/resource/vegetarian-vegan-plant-based-diet.html

7 Weder S, Keller M, Fischer M, Becker K, Alexy U. Intake of micronutrients and fatty acids of vegetarian, vegan, and omnivorous children (1-3 years) in Germany (VeChi Diet Study). Eur J Nutr. 2022; 61(3):1507–20. https://doi.org/10.1007/s00394-021-02753-3.

8 https://foodfoundation.org.uk/sites/default/files/2021-09/Peas-Please-Veg-Facts-2021-Mobile-Friendly.pdf

9 http://healthsurvey.hscic.gov.uk/media/1092/_7-fruit-and-vegetable-consumption_7th-proof.pdf

10 https://commonslibrary.parliament.uk/research-briefings/sn03336/

11 Koletzko B, Godfrey KM, Poston L, Szajewska H, van Goudoever JB, de Waard M, et al. Nutrition during pregnancy, lactation and early childhood and its implications for maternal and long-term child health: the early nutrition project recommendations. Ann Nutr Metab. 2019;74(2):93–106. https://doi.org/10.1159/000496471.

12 Günther ALB, Remer T, Kroke A, Buyken AE. Early protein intake and later obesity risk: which protein sources at which time points throughout infancy and childhood are important for body mass index and body fat percentage at 7 y of age? Am J Clin Nutr. 2007;86(6):1765–72. https://doi.org/10.1093/ajcn/86.5.1765.

13 Sabaté J, Wien M. Vegetarian diets and childhood obesity prevention. Am J Clin Nutr. 2010;91(5): 1525S–9S. https://doi.org/10.3945/ajcn.2010.28701F.
14 Carbohydrate and Health. Scientific Advisory Committee on Nutrition. 2015. Published by TSO (The Stationery Office) and Available from: www.tsoshop.co.uk
15 Alexy U, Fischer M, Weder S, Längler A, Michalsen A, Sputtek A, et al. Nutrient intake and status of German children and adolescents consuming vegetarian, vegan or omnivore diets: results of the VeChi youth study. Nutrients. 2021;13(5):1707. https://doi.org/10.3390/nu13051707.
16 Fleischer DM, Chan ES, Venter C, Spergel JM, Abrams EM, Stukus D, et al. A consensus approach to the primary prevention of food allergy through nutrition: guidance from the American Academy of Allergy, Asthma, and Immunology; American College of Allergy, Asthma, and Immunology; and the Canadian Society for Allergy and Clinical Immunology. J Allergy Clin Immunol Pract. 2021;9(1):22–43.e4. https://doi.org/10.1016/j.jaip.2020.11.002.
17 Logan K, Bahnson HT, Ylescupidez A, Beyer K, Bellach J, Campbell DE, et al. Early introduction of peanut reduces peanut allergy across risk groups in pooled and causal inference analyses. Allergy. 2023;78(5):1307–18. https://doi.org/10.1111/all.15597.
18 Du Toit G, Roberts G, Sayre PH, Bahnson HT, Radulovic S, Santos AF, et al. Randomized trial of peanut consumption in infants at risk for peanut allergy. N Engl J Med. 2015;372(9):803–13. https://doi.org/10.1056/NEJMoa1414850.
19 Perkin MR, Logan K, Marrs T, Radulovic S, Craven J, Flohr C, et al. Enquiring About Tolerance (EAT) study: feasibility of an early allergenic food introduction regimen. J Allergy Clin Immunol. 2016; 137(5):1477–86.e8. https://doi.org/10.1016/j.jaci.2015.12.1322.
20 Togias A, Cooper SF, Acebal ML, Assa'ad A, Baker JR Jr, Beck LA, et al. Addendum guidelines for the prevention of peanut allergy in the United States: report of the National Institute of Allergy and Infectious Diseases-sponsored expert panel. J Allergy Clin Immunol. 2017;139(1):29–44. https://doi.org/10.1016/j.jaci.2016.10.010.
21 Department of Health. Dietary Reference Values for Food Energy and Nutrients for the United Kingdom. HMSO; 1991.
22 Uauy R, Dangour AD. Fat and fatty acid requirements and recommendations for infants of 0-2 years and children of 2-18 years. Ann Nutr Metab. 2009;55(1-3):76–96. https://doi.org/10.1159/000228997.
23 https://plantbasedhealthprofessionals.com/wp-content/uploads/Factsheet_-Feeding-your-vegan-baby-8.pdf
24 https://plantbasedhealthprofessionals.com/wp-content/uploads/Factsheet-Feeding-your-vegan-babyThe-second-Year-Final.pdf
25 Gardner CD, Hartle JC, Garrett RD, Offringa LC, Wasserman AS. Maximizing the intersection of human health and the health of the environment with regard to the amount and type of protein produced and consumed in the United States. Nutr Rev. 2019;77(4):197–215. https://doi.org/10.1093/nutrit/nuy073.
26 Mariotti F, Gardner CD. Dietary protein and amino acids in vegetarian diets-a review. Nutrients. 2019;11(11):2661. https://doi.org/10.3390/nu11112661.
27 Friel J, Qasem W, Cai C. Iron and the breastfed infant. Antioxidants (Basel). 2018;7(4):54. https://doi.org/10.3390/antiox7040054.
28 Pawlak R, Bell K. Iron status of vegetarian children: a review of literature. Ann Nutr Metab. 2017; 70(2):88–99. https://doi.org/10.1159/000466706.
29 Desmond MA, Sobiecki JG, Jaworski M, Płudowski P, Antoniewicz J, Shirley MK, et al. Growth, body composition, and cardiovascular and nutritional risk of 5- to 10-y-old children consuming vegetarian, vegan, or omnivore diets. Am J Clin Nutr. 2021;113(6):1565–77. https://doi.org/10.1093/ajcn/nqaa445.
30 Mangels AR. Bone nutrients for vegetarians. Am J Clin Nutr. 2014;100(suppl 1):469S–75S. https://doi.org/10.3945/ajcn.113.071423.
31 Vanderpump MP, Lazarus JH, Smyth PP, Laurberg P, Holder RL, Boelaert K, et al. Iodine status of UK schoolgirls: a cross-sectional survey. Lancet. 2011; 377(9782):2007–12. https://doi.org/10.1016/S0140-6736(11)60693-4.
32 https://www.bda.uk.com/resource/iodine.html
33 Menal-Puey S, Martínez-Biarge M, Marques-Lopes I. Developing a food exchange system for meal planning in vegan children and adolescents. Nutrients. 2018;11(1):43. https://doi.org/10.3390/nu11010043.

Paula Hallam
Plant Based Kids Ltd.
39 Queens Road
Kingston upon Thames KT2 7SL, UK
paula@plantbased-kids.com

Published online: November 15, 2024

Szajewska H, Neu J, Shamir R, Wong G, Prentice AM (eds): Shaping the Future with Nutrition. Nestle Nutr Inst Workshop Ser. Basel, Karger, 2024, vol 100, pp 170–179 (DOI: 10.1159/000540148)

Healthy Diets at the Intersection of Human and Planetary Health

Jose M. Saavedra

Johns Hopkins University School of Medicine, Baltimore, MD, USA

Abstract

Our diets are the greatest determinant of health, and what we eat is sustained and shaped by the food we produce. Food systems have increased production to feed the growing world population, which has also led to a dietary transition, with increases in energy and protein intakes, and only modest improvements in micronutrient density. Thus, undernutrition has decreased globally, while non-communicable diseases are dramatically increasing. Today, food systems are being threatened by global warming. Conversely, food systems are a major contributor to climate change and environmental degradation, generating one-quarter of all greenhouse gasses, using half of the world's habitable land, and are the largest source of water pollution. The greatest contributor to this environmental degradation is the production of animal-based foods, particularly meat. Food systems must ensure access to safe, nutritious, and sustainable foods (e.g., improving yields, reducing waste, and greenhouse gas emissions), decreasing animal-based food production, and increasing plant-based foods, which can positively impact our diets. On the "demand side", shifting our current diets from high animal-based foods to plant-based diets will decrease global mortality and disability. Our diet is at the intersection of our health and our planet's health and, thus, a major instrument to improve both.

Introduction

Foods are those components of the environment that are consumed by animals, and determine their optimal growth, development, and reproduction – the basis for health of all species [1].

Over 300,000 years, *Homo sapiens* learned to modify their environment to support their individual and social food needs, to survive in most ecological niches in the world, and to become the global dominant animal species. This extraordinary achievement was made possible by the relatively recent development of agricultural technology and food systems, which, over the last 10,000 years, allowed humans to multiply in every corner of the earth and expand all aspects of science, technology, and the humanities. This progress has come at a price. The impact of human development, including agriculture, on climate change and other environmental threats is palpable and undeniable. Agriculture and food systems that sustain our diets contribute to climate change. And reciprocally, climate change impacts agricultural outputs and food systems. What we eat and how we produce and procure these foods impact our health and our planet's health.

Diet as a Determinant of Human Health

After slow, steady growth for thousands of years, the population of the world and its nutritional needs have grown exponentially since the beginning of the Industrial Revolution in the 1850s. It took more than 200,000 years for the world population to reach 2 billion, but only 25 years to grow the last 2 billion, to reach 8 billion inhabitants. Nevertheless, we currently produce enough food to feed all inhabitants, albeit unequally distributed. The food we produce and eat today, our diets, directly correlate with the state of health of the world's population.

The last 150 years saw dramatic decreases in infant and adult mortality and morbidity, mainly from infectious disease and malnutrition. Over the last 50 years, we saw huge decreases in infant mortality, by more than 60%, and in childhood stunting, by more than 70%, with dramatic decreases in micronutrient deficiencies, particularly iodine and vitamin A. However, to date, 22% of the world's children under 5 years of age remain stunted, almost 7% of children have wasting, and at least half of the children under 5 have single or multiple micronutrient deficiencies.

In the last decade, progress towards decreasing undernutrition has slowed down, and this has been exacerbated by the recent COVID-19 pandemic. Moreover, the distribution of this progress has been very uneven – 94% of all stunted children and 97% of all children with wasting live in Asia and Africa. At the other end of the spectrum, obesity has increased in every country in the world and has tripled since 1975. Today, 39% of adults over 18 are overweight and 13% are obese. Childhood obesity under 5 is around 7% of all children, and more than 85% of them live in Asia or Africa. In absolute numbers, it is expected that child and adolescent obesity will have surpassed moderate or severe underweight in the last 2 years [2, 3].

Changes in nutrition mirror the rise of non-communicable diseases (NCDs). Cardiovascular disease, diabetes, chronic respiratory disease, and cancer are now responsible for 65% of all disability, or healthy life years lost to disease. Global deaths from NCDs have increased from 61% of all deaths (31 million) in 2000 to 74% (41 million) in 2019. More than 75% of deaths occur in low- and middle-income countries [4]. This underlies the trends in risk factors for death and disability. In 2010, child wasting, low birth weight, and prematurity were the top three leading risk factors for disability. Today they are the 11th, 4th, and 22nd in ranking. On the other hand, high blood pressure, high fasting plasma glucose, high body mass index, and high low-density lipoprotein (LDL) cholesterol are all in the top 8 risk factors for disability, and they are the fastest-increasing risks for death and disability [5].

These changes are the result of what we eat, as the world has undergone a global dietary transition. Energy intakes remained stable for more than 200 years. However, driven by changes in technology and the global food system, starting in high-income countries in the 1960s and 70s, energy supply and intake increased significantly, while physical energy expenditure decreased. This "flipping point" began in high-income countries, is now global, and is responsible for the epidemic of obesity and NCDs [6]. These increases reflect the increase in overweight and obesity as well as their disparate distribution. The average global supply of calories per person increased by about 700 kcal/d, with widely different increases of approximately 500 kcal/d in Africa (to reach 2,200 kcal/d), 740 kcal/d in North America (to reach 3,500 kcal/d), and a staggering 2,000 kcal/d increase in China (to now 3,400 kcal/d). Forty-eight percent of the world eats either too many or too few calories [7].

The global state of nutrition reflects the changes in energy intake and the foods that comprise overall diets. Today, no world region meets the recommendation for the intake of key foods. Globally, the intake of fruits, legumes, and whole grains is only 40%, and vegetables only 60%, of what is recommended. Intakes of legumes and nuts fair worse, around 25% to 30% of recommended intakes. On the other hand, intake of starchy vegetables and eggs is generally higher than recommended. Red meat intake is 500% above recommendations, with high average per capita intakes even in low and middle-income countries [8, 9].

The Global Burden of Disease is a comprehensive study of global mortality and disability, which identified dietary risks as the second highest risk factor for global mortality, second only to high systolic blood pressure in females, and third to high blood pressure and smoking in males. Six of the top ten risk factors for global mortality from NCDs (high BP, poor diet, high plasma glucose, high BMI, high LDL cholesterol, and poor child maternal nutrition) are diet related. In the aggregate, suboptimal diets are responsible for more deaths than any other risks globally, including tobacco smoking. The leading dietary risk factors for mortality are diets high in sodium, sugar, and sweetened beverages, red meat, and trans fats; and low in whole grains, fruit, vegetables, nuts, seeds, and omega-3 fatty acids [5, 10].

Interdependency of Diet and Food Systems

Until 8–10,000 years ago, food was gathered, and animals were hunted. Agriculture, the production of food from the land, led to a surplus for consumption, allowing extensive and complex societal groups to emerge. Technologies for conserving, transporting, and distributing food gave rise to what we call today "food systems" or "agri-food systems," which became truly global following the Industrial Revolution. Agri-food systems include all elements and interconnections associated with the production of food and non-food products (from crops, livestock, fisheries, forestry, and aquaculture), the food supply chain from producer to consumer (production, processing, distribution and marketing, preparation) and the final consumption of food and its waste and disposal, including socio-economic and environmental outcomes [11, 12].

Since the 1960s, technology allowed dramatic increases in global food production, increasing agricultural land use, but mainly through more efficient land use. In just the last 50 years, global cereal production tripled, increasing 150% in North America, 500% in China, and 700% in Brazil. Global dairy production increased by 270%, cane sugar by 350%, meat by 500%, and soy 13 times (1,300%) [13]. In global numbers, this kept up with the additional 5 billion growth in population and with the global GDP, which grew 800% [14].

Globally, there was greater food availability, affordability, and consequently greater consumption. With wide regional variations, the global per capita energy supply increased by about 700 kcal/d since 1960. Per capita protein supply increased by 22 g/d and fat by 40 g/d. Increases in intake per capita over this period occurred in every world region, but the amount of increase strongly correlated to per capita GDP. Not only has energy and protein supply and consumption increased, but with increased economic growth, diets have shifted from protein from plant sources to a greater protein intake from animal foods. From 1960 to 2020, the global per capita animal protein supply increased by 50% (from 20 g to 33 g). In high-income countries, 60% of total protein consumed is from animal sources, mostly meat. In low-income countries, only 15% of protein comes from animal sources [7, 13].

Changes in the global food system, particularly reductions in the time-cost of food, and greater acquisition power, appear as major drivers of global dietary changes and the rise of obesity. This dietary transition is global, with major differences depending on region, country, and socioeconomic development. In addition, mechanization, urbanization, motorization, and digital media environments contribute to decreasing energy expenditures. Finally, the proliferation, availability, low cost, and commercial promotion of energy-dense, high-sugar, and high-sodium foods 'feeds an increasing demand and decreases diet quality. Food systems are globally contributing to poor diet quality and obesogenic environments [6, 15].

Despite these changes, today, 5.4% of the world population can still not afford a calorie-sufficient diet, 31% cannot afford a nutrient-sufficient diet, and 42% (3.3 billion) cannot afford a healthy diet [7]. Inadequate agricultural subsidies, work and labor dependencies, inappropriate marketing, and poor consumer information and education, all affect food systems, food security, and shape our diets.

It is clear that while our food systems have sustained the world population and decreased hunger, they have yet to resolve growing inequities and have contributed to an undesirable dietary transition with major health consequences. Progress in science and technology has enabled the capability of producing food for eight billion inhabitants. However, current food systems are falling short. Furthermore, these systems are now threatened by environmental changes, which may worsen global nutrition and health inequities and be insufficient to keep up with continued population growth.

Reciprocal Impact between Food Systems and Planet Health

Climate Affects Food Systems

Since the industrialization of the 1850s, the average temperature of the planet has increased by more than 1°C. Human emissions of greenhouse gases are the primary driver of this rapid increase. Unchecked, temperature rises at or above 1.5°C will not only increase the frequency of extreme weather events (heat waves, droughts, storms, and floods), as we are now experiencing, but will significantly increase sea level rise and have long-lasting effects on our environment for centuries or millennia. Climate change severely threatens the environment's future and profoundly affects the biosphere, plants, animals, and human society [16]. These environmental changes will drastically affect not only wildlife but also the plant and animal outputs that sustain our current food systems.

Extreme weather events disrupt water systems, and rising sea levels can decrease crop yields and productivity in livestock and fisheries. There is strong evidence that climate change will affect food quality through decreased diversity and nutrient density. Elevated CO_2 is associated with reduced concentrations of zinc, iron, and protein, particularly in wheat, rice, and maize, the world's largest sources of calories [17, 18]. Climate also affects the ability to produce, move, and distribute food, decreasing food availability, access, and affordability. Impacts on food storage, processing, transportation, and on water systems can increase foodborne pathogens and mycotoxins, affecting food safety. Overall, climate change significantly affects food security, and the negative impact disproportionally affects low- and middle-income countries. Some place the impact at more than 500,000 additional deaths between 2010 and 2050 due to climate-related diet changes [17, 19, 20].

Food Systems Affect Climate

Conversely, current food systems negatively affect the environment and are major contributors to climate change. The food that makes up our diets today is responsible for one-quarter of greenhouse gas (GHG) emissions contributing to global warming. Agricultural land use and food production, processing, packaging, and food waste emit similar amounts of GHG to global electricity and heat production, and almost double the GHG emissions from transportation.

Which foods we produce makes a difference. Of all the emissions from food production, 31% come from livestock and fisheries (animals raised for meat, dairy, eggs, and seafood). Most of these gasses are methane and CO2 from the digestive processes of cattle and their manure. Of the foods we consume, GHG emissions for plant products are 10 to 50 times lower than for animal products. Red meat is by far the highest contributor to GHG, producing more than 2× the GHG per kg of lamb, more than 10× that of fish or eggs, and more than 50 to 60× the GHG from wheat, maize, fruits, and vegetables. On average, producing animal protein (meat and dairy) requires 11 times more fossil fuel energy than grain-based protein. Red meat production is especially inefficient; the estimated ratio of kcal of energy used to kcal of protein generated in meat production is 57:1 for lamb and 40:1 for beef. This effect is compounded by the fact that less than half – only 48% – of the world's production of cereals is eaten by humans. Today, about 40% of cereal crops are used for animal feed, and 11% for biofuels [19, 21].

In addition, food systems contribute to other environmental threats to planet health. About 20 years ago, the UN endorsed the concept of planetary boundaries: specific "ecological ceilings" past which there is a risk of large-scale, abrupt, or irreversible environmental changes to the planet [22]. These key measures of planet health include climate change and land use, as well as biodiversity loss and extinctions, nitrogen and phosphorus pollution of the biosphere and oceans, ocean acidification, and freshwater consumption.

Food systems significantly impact these planet health boundaries. Food production uses 50% of the world's habitable land, of which 77% is for raising livestock. Only 23% of agricultural land is used for crops for human consumption, providing 82% of calories and 63% of dietary protein consumed. Food systems produce 26% of all GHG, use 70% of fresh water, and cause 78% of water pollution (mainly from nitrogen and phosphates from fertilizer and animal waste). Wild animals are becoming extinct, and biodiversity is decreasing at unprecedented rates. While difficult to fathom, of the global bird biomass, 71% is poultry livestock, and only 29% are wild birds. And outside humans, 94% of the global biomass of mammals is livestock for human consumption. Only 4% of global mammal biomass are wild mammals [21].

The Need for Change and Today's Opportunities

Our diet is the greatest determinant of global health. Our current calorie intake and dietary choices are far from ideal and will require a significant change to improve global health. And the food systems that shape our diets today not only drive inadequate intake but are themselves driven by our food choices. Furthermore, the food systems that support today's food supply are being *affected by* and are *contributing to* climate change and other environmental threats to our planet. These interactions are major determinants of the state of human and planet health, and thus also represent a major opportunity.

Slowing down global warming, among other human activities, will require a change in our food systems and dietary habits. Fortunately, there are synergies in attaining these goals. The foods associated with lower health risks (fruits, vegetables, legumes, whole grain cereals, and nuts) are also associated with lower environmental impacts. On the other hand, aside from the overall excess in calorie intake, foods associated with the most significant increases in morbidity and mortality (processed and unprocessed meat) are associated with the greatest negative environmental impact. Shifting our current diets from high amounts of animal-based foods to increasingly healthier plant-based diets can decrease land use, greenhouse gas emissions, freshwater use, and water pollution, and at the same time, reduce risks of NCDs. Sustainable food systems can reciprocally promote sustainable, healthier diets and benefit human and planet health – a win-win situation [9, 15, 23].

On the "demand side" of the equation, global diets must shift to more sustainable consumption patterns. This will require adopting a plant-rich diet with moderate amounts of dairy, eggs, and meat. Examples are the Mediterranean diet and specific recommendations such as the planetary health "EAT" diet proposed by The Lancet Commission. It will also require adjusting global per capita caloric intake to healthier levels, e.g., 2,100 calories per day. Care will need to be taken to adapt levels regionally and to specific vulnerable populations, including young children and pregnant women [20, 24, 25].

On the "supply side," food systems must ensure access to safe and nutritious food for all and increase "nature-positive production at scale" by adopting practices that protect and restore ecosystems. Among other things, this will require achieving higher agricultural yields, including improving crop genetics and agronomic practices. It will also require reducing food waste, GHG emissions, and polluting effects of foods, by increasing production efficiency (e.g., altering precise use of nitrogen fertilizers and additives to nutrient ruminant feed). Some analysis indicates that staying within planetary boundaries is possible, but will require action in all aspects of food production [24, 26].

Implementing these changes will not be simple or easy, but will be necessary. This will require participation of all sectors of society to ensure these changes are realized fairly and equitably, tailored to social, political, economic, and cultural values. Multiple interdisciplinary efforts are underway, identifying solutions and approaches to meeting these goals – intrinsically related to the UN's sustainable development goals for 2030. The latest UN Food Systems Summit in 2021 acknowledged that sustainable food production systems should be recognized as an essential solution to these challenges – to feed a growing global population while protecting our planet. "Food is the single strongest lever to optimize human health and environmental sustainability on Earth" [25, 27].

Social and political leadership are critical to these goals. However, everyone can play a role, particularly, those engaged in the healthcare and nutrition sectors. There is an increasing awareness of the relationship between food, health, and the environment, particularly in younger generations, which can be leveraged to implement these changes. Education at every level to increase the demand of foods for a healthier diet should be seen not only as a path to better health for people, their families, and their communities but as a way to build a healthier planet. Our diet is at the intersection of human and planetary health. It is, therefore, an effective instrument to improve both.

Conflict of Interest Statement

The author has no conflicts of interest to declare. The author received lecture honoraria and travel reimbursement from Nestlé Nutrition Institute.

References

1 Hartenstein V, Martinez P. Structure, development and evolution of the digestive system. Cell Tissue Res. 2019;377(3):289–92. https://doi.org/10.1007/s00441-019-03102-x.

2 UNICEF, WHO, The World Bank. Levels and Trends in Child Malnutrition: Key Findings of the 2021 Edition of the Joint Child Malnutrition Estimates. Geneva: World Health Organization; 2021.

3 NCD Risk Factor Collaboration (NCD-RisC). Worldwide trends in body-mass index, underweight, overweight, and obesity from 1975 to 2016: a pooled analysis of 2416 population-based measurement studies in 128.9 million children, adolescents, and adults. Lancet. 2017;390(10113):2627–42. https://doi.org/10.1016/S0140-6736(17)32129-3.

4 World Health Organization (WHO). Global health estimates September 2023. Online resource accessed November 10, 2023. Available from: https://www.who.int/news-room/fact-sheets/detail/noncommunicable-diseases.

5 GBD 2019 Risk Factors Collaborators. Global burden of 87 risk factors in 204 countries and territories, 1990-2019: a systematic analysis for the Global Burden of Disease Study 2019. Lancet. 2020;396(10258):1223–49. https://doi.org/10.1016/S0140-6736(20)30752-2.

6 Swinburn BA, Sacks G, Hall KD, McPherson K, Finegood DT, Moodie ML, et al. The global obesity pandemic: shaped by global drivers and local environments. Lancet. 2011;378(9793):804–14. https://doi.org/10.1016/S0140-6736(11)60813-1.

7 Roser M, Ritchie H, Rosado P. Food supply. 2013. Published online at: OurWorldInData.org Based on FAO data, updated to 2020. Online resource accessed November 10, 2023. Available from: https://ourworldindata.org/food-supply.

8 Global Nutrition Report 2021. The State of Global Nutrition. Bristol, UK: Development Initiatives; 2021.

9 Willett W, Rockström J, Loken B, Springmann M, Lang T, Vermeulen S, et al. Food in the Anthropocene: the EAT-Lancet Commission on healthy diets from sustainable food systems. Lancet. 2019;393(10170):447–92. https://doi.org/10.1016/S0140-6736(18)31788-4.

10 GBD 2017 Diet Collaborators. Health effects of dietary risks in 195 countries, 1990-2017: a systematic analysis for the Global Burden of Disease Study 2017. Lancet. 2019;393(10184):1958–72. https://doi.org/10.1016/S0140-6736(19)30041-8. Erratum in: Lancet. 2021;397(10293):2466.

11 United Nations (UN). Final report by the Zero hunger challenge working groups, Advisory note for action - all food systems are sustainable. High level Task Force of Global Food and Nutrition Security entities. FAO, UNCTAD, UNIDO, World Bank. 2015. Online resource accessed November 10, 2023. Available from: https://www.un.org/en/issues/food/taskforce/pdf/ZHC%20ANs-%20All%20Merged%20Rev%20May%202016.pdf.

12 Food and Agriculture Organization (FAO). The State of Food and Agriculture 2021. Making Agrifood Systems More Resilient to Shocks and Stresses. Rome: FAO; 2021. Online resource accessed November 10, 2023. Available from: https://doi.org/10.4060/cb4476en.

13 Ritchie H, Rosado P, Roser M. Agricultural production. 2023. Published online at: OurWorldInData.org. Online resource accessed November 10, 2023. Available from: https://ourworldindata.org/agricultural-production

14 World Bank national accounts data, and OECD National Accounts data files. GDP 2023. Online resource accessed November 10, 2023. Available from: https://data.worldbank.org/indicator/NY.GDP.MKTP.KD.

15 Hemler EC, Hu FB. Plant-based diets for personal, population, and planetary health. Adv Nutr. 2019;10(suppl 1_4):S275–83. https://doi.org/10.1093/advances/nmy117.

16 Intergovernmental Panel on Climate Change (IPCC). 2018: Summary for policymakers. In: Masson-Delmotte V, Zhai P, Pörtner HO, Roberts D, Skea J, Shukla PR, et al, eds. Global Warming of 1.5°C. An IPCC Special Report on the impacts of global warming of 1.5°C above pre-industrial levels and related global greenhouse gas emission pathways, in the context of strengthening the global response to the threat of climate change, sustainable development, and efforts to eradicate poverty. Cambridge, UK and New York, NY, USA: Cambridge University Press; 2018, pp. 3–24. https://doi.org/10.1017/9781009157940.001.

17 Fanzo J, Davis C, McLaren R, Choufani J. The effect of climate change across food systems: implications for nutrition outcomes. Global Food Secur. 2018;18:12–9. https://doi.org/10.1016/j.gfs.2018.06.001.

18 Myers SS, Zanobetti A, Kloog I, Huybers P, Leakey AD, Bloom AJ, et al. Increasing CO2 threatens human nutrition. Nature. 2014;510(7503):139–42. https://doi.org/10.1038/nature13179.
19 Intergovernmental Panel on Climate Change (IPCC). Summary for policymakers. In: Climate Change and Land: IPCC Special Report on Climate Change, Desertification, Land Degradation, Sustainable Land Management, Food Security, and Greenhouse Gas Fluxes in Terrestrial Ecosystems. Cambridge: Cambridge University Press; 2022, pp. 1–36.
20 Springmann M, Clark M, Mason-D'Croz D, Wiebe K, Bodirsky BL, Lassaletta L, et al: Options for keeping the food system within environmental limits. Nature. 2018;562(7728):519–25. https://doi.org/10.1038/s41586-018-0594-0.
21 Ritchie H, Rosado P, Roser M. Environmental impacts of food production. 2022. Published online at: OurWorldInData.org. Online resource accessed November 10, 2023. Available from: https://ourworldindata.org/environmental-impacts-of-food.
22 Richardson K, Steffen W, Lucht W, Bendtsen J, Cornell SE, Donges JF, et al. Earth beyond six of nine planetary boundaries. Sci Adv. 2023;9(37): eadh2458. https://doi.org/10.1126/sciadv.adh2458.
23 Clark MA, Springmann M, Hill J, Tilman D. Multiple health and environmental impacts of foods. Proc Natl Acad Sci U S A 2019;116(46): 23357–62. https://doi.org/10.1073/pnas.1906908116.
24 Clark MA, Domingo NGG, Colgan K, Thakrar SK, Tilman D, Lynch J, et al. Global food system emissions could preclude achieving the 1.5° and 2°C climate change targets. Science. 2020; 370(6517):705–8. https://doi.org/10.1126/science.aba7357.
25 United Nations. Secretary-general's chair summary and statement of action on the UN food systems summit. Food Systems Summit 2021. Online resource accessed November 10, 2023. Available from: https://www.un.org/en/food-systems-summit.
26 Springmann M, Wiebe K, Mason-D'Croz D, Sulser TB, Rayner M, Scarborough P. Health and nutritional aspects of sustainable diet strategies and their association with environmental impacts: a global modelling analysis with country-level detail. Lancet Planet Health. 2018; 2(10):e451–61. https://doi.org/10.1016/S2542-5196(18)30206-7.
27 The EAT-lancet commission on food, planet, health. EAT-lancet commission summary report. Online resource accessed November 10, 2023. Available from: https://eatforum.org/eat-lancet-commission/eat-lancet-commission-summary-report/.

Jose M. Saavedra
Department of Pediatrics
Johns Hopkins University School of Medicine
6 Beekman Place
Morristown, NJ 07960 USA
jose@saavedra.pe

Published online: November 15, 2024

Szajewska H, Neu J, Shamir R, Wong G, Prentice AM (eds): Shaping the Future with Nutrition. Nestle Nutr Inst Workshop Ser. Basel, Karger, 2024, vol 100, pp 180–191 (DOI: 10.1159/000540151)

New Food Technologies – Addressing Challenges at Food Systems Level

Julia K. Keppler[a] David L. Kaplan[b] Marine R.-C. Kraus[c]

[a]Laboratory of Food Process Engineering, Wageningen University and Research, Wageningen, The Netherlands; [b]Department of Biomedical Engineering, Tufts University, Medford, MA, USA; [c]Nestlé Research, Nestlé Institute of Health Sciences, Lausanne, Switzerland

Abstract

By 2050, the global population is expected to reach close to 10 billion people, increasing the demand for food. To ensure sustainability in food production to meet this population increase, alternative approaches such as reducing meat consumption and incorporating plant-based alternatives are being explored. Cellular agriculture, an interdisciplinary field merging engineering and biology offers a potential solution. This approach involves the isolation and modification of animal cells for food production, using techniques like genetic engineering and creating cell-biomaterial interfaces. This approach has the potential to provide sustainable and nutritious meat and dairy alternatives while reducing environmental impact. However, challenges such as achieving the same nutritional quality and texture as animal-based products and addressing issues related to scale-up as well as costs pose barriers to commercialization. Despite these challenges, cellular agriculture has progressed rapidly and shows promise in meeting the changing demands of consumers and ensuring food security in the future.

Introduction

By 2050, the global population is expected to hit close to 10 billion people. The ever-growing human population will substantially increase the demand for food and compels consideration of alternative approaches toward food sustainability, nutrition, and security [1]. The transition to a sustainable food system requires the reduction in consumption of meat and fish products, and plant-based alternatives have emerged as an option. However, plant-based proteins such as soy or pea may not have matching nutritional quality and have technical limitations regarding texture challenges and sensory properties. Alternatively, cellular agriculture may allow the production of meat and fish products with matching protein quality to its animal-produced tissues. Hence the food industry is constantly evolving, and new technologies are emerging to meet the changing demands of consumers.

Cellular agriculture, also known as cell culture-based food production, offers a potential alternative to conventional farming methods [2]. This innovative approach could reduce the environmental impact associated with traditional agriculture while ensuring high nutritional and sensory quality, ingredient safety, and food security. This is an interdisciplinary field that merges principles from engineering and biology to generate cells for diverse purposes. This field employs cutting-edge techniques such as genetic engineering, biomaterials, and microfabrication to design and modify cells and tissues to match animal products consumed today.

Ten years ago, the first lab-grown beef burger was made from bovine muscle stem cells cultivated to form mature muscle fibers and combined to form a hamburger. Meanwhile, the industry is exploring consumer acceptance, regulatory concerns, and the social, economic, and environmental impact of cellular agriculture. Notably, the FDA has recently granted approval for lab-grown chicken to be consumed by humans [3], and similar techniques could potentially be employed to produce complex milk bioactive that are difficult to obtain through other technologies, like traditional microbial processes.

Transforming the Future of Food with Cellular Agriculture Technologies for Meat Alternatives Development

The development of meat alternatives via cellular agriculture combines a cell-based, tissue engineering approach (cells, scaffolding, feed ingredients, bioreactors), along with the integration of plant-based materials and alternative proteins as components for the process [4]. Sustainable, cost-effective, and scalable cultivated meat and alternative proteins may provide new and nutritious food alternatives while decreasing negative environmental impacts [5]. Towards this goal, key cells, biomaterials, and systems engineering are factors to optimize in the process in order to achieve quality protein-rich foods and match current animal-derived products that consumers prefer. However, many factors must be considered for successful systems integration for cellular agriculture processes and biomanufacturing needs to meet such consumer demands, including the cells, media, biomaterials, and systems.

Over the past few years, significant advances have been realized in many aspects of the field of cellular agriculture for meat production. At the core, cells, most often isolated from tissue biopsies from selected animals, are subsequently expanded and then differentiated to grow into tissues, with a focus on muscle (for texture) and fat (for flavor and taste) (Fig. 1). Cells have been isolated and characterized from livestock sources such as pig, cow, chicken, turkey, and others, as well as from a range of fish [6, 7]. Some of these cells have been immortalized via spontaneous methods (e.g., serum starvation, UV exposure, chemicals), while others have been genetically modified (e.g., transposon, CRISPR) [8, 9]. These immortalization processes are key to generating cell stocks for long-term utility in the field to avoid process variability and to also avoid the need to go back to the host animal for additional cell material collection.

Media costs are most often cited in lifecycle analyses and technoeconomic analyses as the most expensive aspect of cellular agriculture, thus, representing a major challenge to further growth of the field [10]. Yet, in the last few years, significant progress has been made with some of these costs to suggest momentum and cost control. These advances include the removal or reduction of bovine serum albumin from media used in cultivating cells and reducing growth factor requirements, both of which offer sizable reductions in media costs. Serum replacement is critical due to cost, variability in sourcing, and the complication or ethical dilemma in (still) using animal-derived ingredients. Growth factors are most often alternative protein products themselves, thus, reducing their use in media has a major impact on reducing costs and the environmental footprint in terms of sustainability. Recent progress includes substituting low-cost agricultural waste extracts, as well as genetically engineered animal cells to reduce both serum requirements and the need for exogenous growth factor additions in media [11].

Cellular agriculture also requires the use of biomaterials which play a key role in many aspects of cell growth and differentiation processes, from scaffolding to support cells in 3D meat-like structures, to cell carriers in bioreactors to enhance cell numbers, to media ingredients derived from extracted or digested low-cost raw material sources (e.g., plant, marine, microbial) [12]. The design and

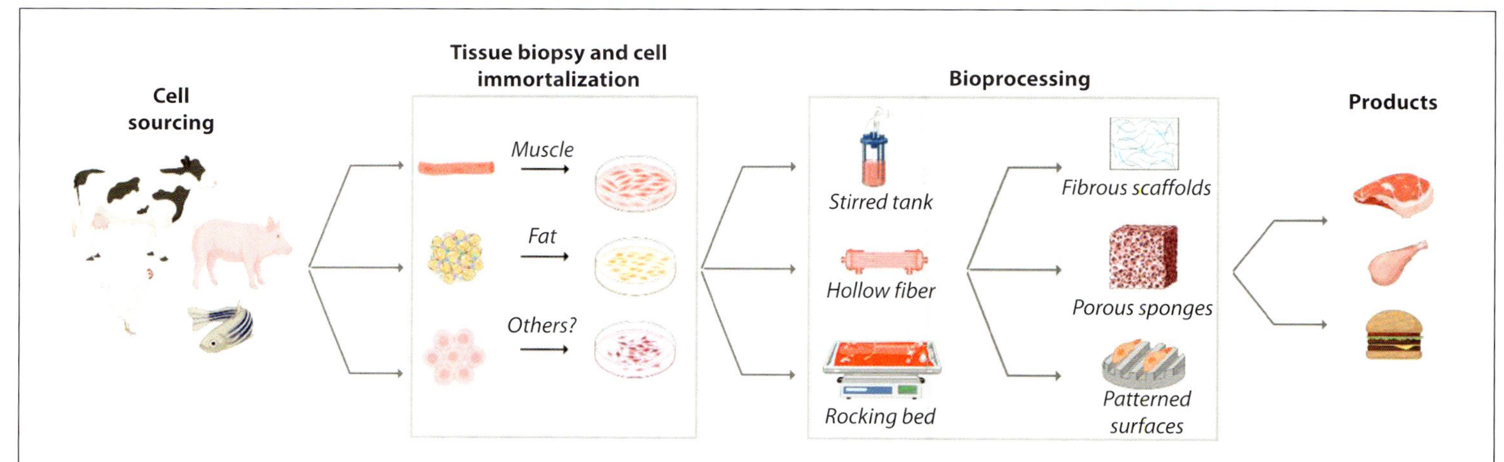

Fig. 1. Non-dairy cellular agriculture products. A cell-culture-based approach is utilized for non-dairy products, where somatic cells from animals, such as skeletal muscle or adipose-progenitor cells, are immortalized and differentiated into the desired tissue lineages. Bioprocessing involves expanding relevant cell types in a bioreactor to generate a large quantity of cells for expansion and differentiation. Bioprinting techniques are employed to mature target cells within on customized, biocompatible tissue scaffolds that support cellular maturation and provide structure and texture to the cultivated product. This figure was created with BioRender.com.

engineering of biomaterials must encompass various aspects to ensure they meet the specific requirements of cells. This includes tailoring surface properties, form factor or morphology (such as films or sponges), and chemistry that facilitates cell binding. This material design and engineering must be accomplished in a sustainable fashion with cost in mind; thus, abundant, low-cost, and available supply chains for biomaterials are key in order to support the scale and needs for cultivated meat into the future.

Scale-up for cell cultivation and cellular agriculture processes, in general, remains an unmet need. There are new efforts to re-design more traditional stirred tank bioreactors to match the needs for cell culture scaling and food production requirements, with an eye toward reduced energy consumption. Significant further innovation is required here to identify scalable and cost-effective approaches. The infrastructure for such scale-up systems still needs to be designed and built, thus, a large gap remains between current research innovation and commercial development to meet the required scale for these future foods. Consequent advancements have been made in the development of bioreactor designs within academic laboratories and start-up companies, indicating progress in this area. Additionally, certain countries have made substantial investments to meet the infrastructure requirements for this technology. However, there is still substantial work to be done in order to achieve the necessary scales for the widespread implementation and growth of this emerging technology.

Aside from the cells, media, biomaterials, and bioreactors, the overall product profile, from taste, flavor, and texture, as well as from safety and regulatory needs is actively being addressed [13, 14]. For example, a number of companies have gained approval for their cellular agriculture products in Singapore and the United States, with others following. However, it is important to note that there are also certain countries or American states where this new technology is met with skepticism or resistance. Further assurance of safety, nutrition, and taste quality, as well as with a view towards a positive impact on the workforce for new jobs and resource incomes may help to further grow the field and open new markets. The current rate of progress, balanced against the growing need for alternative protein-rich foods like meats, will continue to drive this new technology forward for positive impact on consumers.

Cellular Agriculture's Impact on Dairy Alternatives

The field of cellular agriculture is expanding beyond the production of animal-based products like meat, poultry, and seafood to also include dairy alternatives such as milk. Indeed, cellular agriculture may provide a promising alternative to traditional farming for the sustainable production of specific foods, nutrients, and specialized components, including milk-derived products (e.g. cheese) or milk bioactives.

Unlocking the Potential of Precision Fermentation for Milk Protein Production
A way of producing, for instance, milk proteins in vitro is using genetically modified non-animal host cells cultivated in a fermenter. These cells, which can be fungi, bacteria, or yeast, are engineered to produce the desired milk protein, with the host organism being excluded from the final product (Fig. 2). This technology is known as precision fermentation and has been used for more than 40 years to produce valuable bioactive molecules such as insulin or enzymes for food production and detergents [15]. The use of this technology for relatively inexpensive food proteins as a bulk ingredient that is consumed in large quantities has now become almost economically feasible due to technological progress. However, most of the current methods for producing animal-free food proteins are still based on established biotechnological processes. In order to make animal-free food proteins feasible, additional considerations are required [16].

Although these animal-free milk proteins (also called recombinant proteins) offer valuable food proteins without relying on animals, their physical functionality will have to be assessed as they may differ from animal-derived milk proteins due to minor amino acid sequence changes, incorrect folding or lack of glycation or phosphorylation [17]. This in turn could alter their properties as food ingredients, which could affect the ability to obtain a similar texture to animal-based products. However, the use of these recombinant proteins as techno-functional ingredients in animal-free dairy products like cheese poses additional challenges in recreating protein structures and incorporating non-animal fat sources and nutrients. The dominant protein structures responsible for the unique texture of cheese, for example, are casein micelles. Micelles are spherical protein aggregates with a diameter of 200 nm, which are based on intricate interactions between the four different types of casein, calcium, and phosphate [18]. It is extremely difficult to rebuild these structures with potentially misfolded caseins produced by precision fermentation [19, 20]. Furthermore, new technologies need to be developed to either produce such micelles continuously and on a large scale [21] or to find ways to produce cheese structures without micelles.

In addition to dairy products, bioactive milk proteins such as lactoferrin or even milk oligosaccharides can also be produced by precision fermentation. Lactoferrin is a bioactive nutrient with potential benefits for infant nutrition. However, its digestibility and bioactivity need to be established, considering the

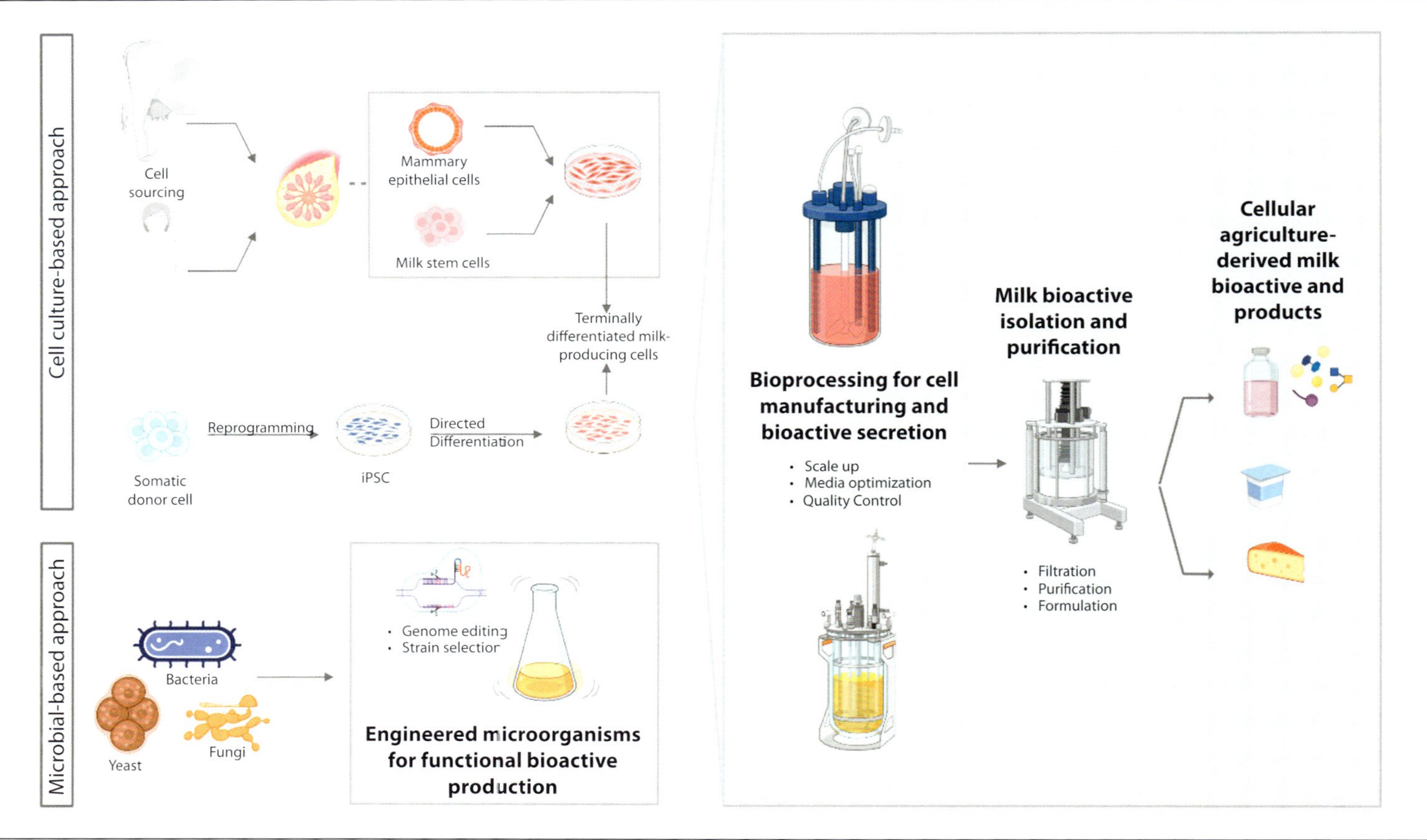

Fig. 2. Dairy cellular agriculture products. Microbial and cell culture approaches are advanced techniques which can be applied for milk bioactive production. Different sources of cells including biopsy-derived mammary epithelial cells, milk stem cells, or even somatic cells, can be utilized to generate terminally differentiated milk-producing cells. Microorganisms such as bacteria, yeast, and fungi can be genetically modified to produce a variety of bioactives found in human milk, including human milk oligosaccharides (HMOs) and human milk proteins (HMPs). The production of milk bioactives and milk-derived products on an industrial scale involves cultivating genetically engineered microorganisms or terminally differentiated milk-producing cells in bioreactors and subsequently purifying them using advanced bioprocessing techniques. This figure was created with BioRender.com.

potential structural differences. Recombinant production of lactoferrin presents an opportunity to produce these bioactive proteins in large quantities, as they are only present in small amounts in animal-based cow milk, and extracting them from milk is a labor-intensive process. It would also be possible to produce human lactoferrin instead of bovine protein, which could be of interest for use in infant formulas.

Finally, to make animal-free milk proteins economically viable, alternative production processes must be established. For example, the extraction of protein from the bioreactor or fermenter still primarily follows biotechnological protocols that were developed for extracting enzymes and bioactive molecules (e.g., protein drugs) with a purity of >90%. However, this purity may not be necessary for use in food. The presence of cell wall polysaccharides in the fermentation broth from the milk-protein-producing host cells such as yeast or fungi might even contribute to ingredient functionality [22, 23]. Current research is therefore investigating the possibility of less intensive purification, which would significantly reduce the processing effort and costs and at the same time improve the ecological footprint of the process [23]. Before scaling up the production of less purified milk proteins obtained through cellular agriculture and precision fermentation, it is crucial to conduct thorough testing for safety, potential off-flavors, and color. These processes are currently being developed in close collaboration with safety and sensory analyses, ensuring a comprehensive evaluation. It is essential to exercise caution and careful evaluation to fully unlock the potential of cellular agriculture and precision fermentation for the development of sustainable dairy alternatives.

Next-Generation Milk by Harnessing Cell-Based Technology for Bioactive Production

One potential area of innovation are infant formulas that provide alternative nutrition for infants that cannot be breastfed. The World Health Organization and the United Nations International Children's Emergency Fund advocate for exclusive breastfeeding for the first 6 months after birth and continued up to the age of 2 years, yet global rates remain low [24, 25]. While infant formulas aim to mimic breast milk, the complexity of human milk composition is difficult to transpose, and therefore commercially available formulas are not capable of providing all the benefits of human breast milk. However, through the innovative combination of synthetic biology and precision fermentation, it is now possible to produce milk components like human milk oligosaccharides (HMOs). A group of small carbohydrates, enriched in human milk and present in lower concentrations and diversity in animal milk. Synthetic HMOs have gained approval for use in infant formulas and have shown promising effects on infant well-being, particularly in gastrointestinal health [26]. These advancements suggest that incorporating HMOs with a composition similar to breast milk could offer valuable benefits and open doors for additional human milk bioactive. Nonetheless, mimicking the intricate complexity of human milk using precision fermentation technology still poses significant challenges. The use of organotypic culture, which mimics the intricate physiology of the mammary gland, holds the potential to enable the production of various milk-specific bioactives, including complex vesicles made from numerous components (Fig. 2) [27]. Recent development of primary cultures of mammary gland epithelial cells has paved the way for the creation of an ex vivo lactation system for cell-based milk production. These biotechnology methods typically involve obtaining a small tissue biopsy from a donor and isolating adult stem cells capable of differentiating into mammary gland cells. The aim is to establish an immortalized cell line that continuously regenerates, eliminating the need for further donor samples. An alternative approach is the use of induced pluripotent stem (iPS) cells, first reported in 2006 [28], which have unlimited expansion potential and can differentiate into any cell type. These versatile cells can also be differentiated into mammary gland epithelial cells for the production of milk bioactives using cell culture-based methods. Despite the complexity and time-consuming nature of iPS cell differentiation protocols, as well as the higher cost associated with the reprogramming process compared to isolating primary adult stem cells, iPS cells have distinct advantages. They offer easier expansion and the remarkable ability to generate unlimited quantities of desired cell populations. When combined with the ability to modify genetic and media culture factors, the organotypic technology enables the modeling of mammary gland organogenesis and lactation processes for the secretion of milk bioactive in a dish [27].

However, effectively inducing the production of functional milk bioactives using mammary gland physiology is complex. Cellular models of mammary gland development, including mammary-like organoids derived from iPS cells and primary cells, have been established and have contributed to the development of human milk components [29, 30]. These organoids can partially mimic pregnancy, lactation, and involution, expressing hormone receptors and secreting milk components, but their long-term growth, functional differentiation, and ability to secrete a full range of milk bioactives still need further demonstration. Additionally, reproducing the structural organization and intricate cell interactions within the mammary gland is particularly challenging, yet crucial for its proper functioning.

Subsequently, the selection of suitable bioreactor types becomes crucial for the large-scale production of cell-based milk bioactives. As an example, stirred tank bioreactors offer scalability, making them ideal for large-scale production, while hollow fiber bioreactors mimic the natural structure of the mammary gland, enabling the efficient production of complex bioactives. By carefully choosing the appropriate bioreactor setup for each stage of the process, the production of cell-based milk bioactives can be further optimized. Yet, to successfully commercialize cell culture-based milk bioactive production, it will be necessary to implement cost-reduction strategies such as utilizing alternative sources of cell culture media. Furthermore, it is important to assess the necessity and cost-effectiveness of utilizing pharmaceutical-grade raw materials in light of the introduction of food-grade cell culture media and ingredients for food production. A potential route to explore further reductions in costs could be the use of potential by-products from bioprocessing.

The FDA's recent announcement declaring laboratory-grown chicken developed in bioreactors as safe for consumption represents a significant advancement in the regulation of cell-based products [3]. While there are similarities between cell culture-based milk bioactives and the bioprocessing of cell culture-based meat products, it is crucial to define and standardize labeling, nomenclature, and communication strategies with consumers as regulatory frameworks for new technologies continue to evolve.

As a result, it becomes feasible to envision the production of functional and personalized milk-like products or bioactive components through cell-based approaches, also offering an alternative to traditional dairy farming. Moreover, the supplementation of infant formulas with human-specific milk bioactives generated by microbial-based and/or mammalian cell culture technologies would have the potential to bring infant formula bioactivity closer to that of human milk.

Conclusion

Although cellular agriculture presents a genuine opportunity for sustainable food production, there are several remaining challenges that need to be addressed for the successful development and implementation of these novel food technologies. Factors such as culture media composition, scale-up processes, bioreactor costs, biomass valorization, and energy consumption have a direct impact on the economics of scale, food quality, consumer preferences, and societal acceptance, as well as regulatory framework. These challenges pose significant opportunities for further innovations that will allow cost-effective commercialization of cellular agriculture for meat and milk production. Addressing these issues will contribute to future sustainable food systems [31].

Acknowledgment

The authors acknowledge the contribution of Pr. Eline Van Der Beek in reviewing the manuscript. The figures were created with BioRender.com.

Conflict of Interest Statement

Marine R.-C. Kraus is an employee of the Société des Produits Nestlé S.A. Switzerland.

Funding Sources

J.K. Keppler and D.L. Kaplan received lecture honoraria and travel reimbursement from Nestlé Nutrition Institute.

Author Contributions

All authors contributed to the writing of the manuscript.

References

1 World population prospects: the 2012 revision—highlights and advance tables. 2013.
2 Rischer H, Szilvay GR, Oksman-Caldentey KM. Cellular agriculture—industrial biotechnology for food and materials. Curr Opin Biotechnol. 2020;61: 128–34. https://doi.org/10.1016/j.copbio.2019.12.003.
3 FDA. FDA Completes First Pre-Market Consultation for Human Food Made Using Animal Cell Culture Technology. FDA; 2022. https://wwwfdagov/food/cfsan-constituent-updates/fda-completes-first-pre-market-consultation-human-food-made-using-animal-cell-culture-technology.
4 Post MJ, Levenberg S, Kaplan DL, Genovese N, Fu J, Bryant CJ, et al. Scientific, sustainability and regulatory challenges of cultured meat. Nat Food. 2020;1(7):403–15. https://doi.org/10.1038/s43016-020-0112-z.
5 Stephens N, Di Silvio L, Dunsford I, Ellis M, Glencross A, Sexton A. Bringing cultured meat to market: technical, socio-political, and regulatory challenges in cellular agriculture. Trends Food Sci Technol. 2018;78:155–66. https://doi.org/10.1016/j.tifs.2018.04.010.
6 Rubio NR, Fish KD, Trimmer BA, Kaplan DL. In vitro insect muscle for tissue engineering applications. ACS Biomater Sci Eng. 2019;5(2):1071–82. https://doi.org/10.1021/acsbiomaterials.8b01261.
7 Saad MK, Yuen JSK, Joyce CM, Li X, Lim T, Wolfson TL, et al. Continuous fish muscle cell line with capacity for myogenic and adipogenic-like phenotypes. Sci Rep. 2023;13(1):5098. https://doi.org/10.1038/s41598-023-31822-2.
8 Gratacap RL, Jin YH, Mantsopoulou M, Houston RD. Efficient genome editing in multiple salmonid cell lines using ribonucleoprotein complexes. Mar Biotechnol (NY). 2020; 22(5):717–24. https://doi.org/10.1007/s10126-020-09995-y.
9 Gratacap RL, Regan T, Dehler CE, Martin SAM, Boudinot P, Collet B, et al. Efficient CRISPR/Cas9 genome editing in a salmonid fish cell line using a lentivirus delivery system. BMC Biotechnol. 2020; 20(1):35. https://doi.org/10.1186/s12896-020-00626-x.
10 O'Neill EN, Ansel JC, Kwong GA, Plastino ME, Nelson J, Baar K, et al. Spent media analysis suggests cultivated meat media will require species and cell type optimization. NPJ Sci Food. 2022; 6(1):46. https://doi.org/10.1038/s41538-022-00157-z.
11 Stout AJ, Rittenberg ML, Shub M, Saad MK, Mirliani AB, Dolgin J, et al. A Beefy-R culture medium: replacing albumin with rapeseed protein isolates. Biomaterials. 2023;296:122092. https://doi.org/10.1016/j.biomaterials.2023.122092.

12 Bomkamp C, Musgrove L, Marques DMC, Fernando GF, Ferreira FC, Specht EA. Differentiation and maturation of muscle and fat cells in cultivated seafood: lessons from developmental biology. Mar Biotechnol (NY). 2023;25(1):1–29. https://doi.org/10.1007/s10126-022-10174-4.

13 Simsa R, Yuen J, Stout A, Rubio N, Fogelstrand P, Kaplan DL. Extracellular heme proteins influence bovine myosatellite cell proliferation and the color of cell-based meat. Foods. 2019;8(10):521. https://doi.org/10.3390/foods8100521.

14 Stout AJ, Zhang X, Letcher SM, Rittenberg ML, Shub M, Chai KM, et al. Engineered autocrine signaling eliminates muscle cell FGF2 requirements for cultured meat production. bioRxiv. 2023:2023.04.17.537163. https://doi.org/10.1101/2023.04.17.537163.

15 Colgrave ML, Dominik S, Tobin AB, Stockmann R, Simon C, Howitt CA, et al. Perspectives on future protein production. J Agric Food Chem. 2021;69(50):15076–83. https://doi.org/10.1021/acs.jafc.1c05989.

16 Bijl E, Keppler JK. Lab-grown food? The precision fermentation approach. In: Pyett S, Jenkins W, van Mierlo B, Trindade LM, Welch D, van Zanten H, eds. Our Future Proteins: A Diversity of Perspectives. VU University Press; 2023, pp. 272–81.

17 Keppler JK, Heyse A, Scheidler E, Uttinger MJ, Fitzner L, Jandt U, et al. Towards recombinantly produced milk proteins: physicochemical and emulsifying properties of engineered whey protein beta-lactoglobulin variants. Food Hydrocolloids. 2021;110:106132. https://doi.org/10.1016/j.foodhyd.2020.106132.

18 Hettinga K, Bijl E. Can recombinant milk proteins replace those produced by animals? Curr Opin Biotechnol. 2022;75:102690. https://doi.org/10.1016/j.copbio.2022.102690.

19 Antuma LJ, Steiner I, Garamus VM, Boom RM, Keppler JK. Engineering artificial casein micelles for future food: is casein phosphorylation necessary? Food Res Int. 2023;173(pt 1):113315. https://doi.org/10.1016/j.foodres.2023.113315.

20 Antuma LJ, Steiner I, Garamus VM, Boom RM, Keppler JK. Engineering artificial casein micelles for future food: is casein phosphorylation necessary? Food Res Int. 2023;173(pt 1):113315. https://doi.org/10.1016/j.foodres.2023.113315.

21 Antuma L, Stadler M, Garamus V, Boom R, Keppler J. Casein micelle formation as a calcium phosphate phase separation process: preparation of artificial casein micelles through vacuum evaporation and membrane processes. Innovative Food Sci Emerging Technol. 2024;92:103582. https://doi.org/10.1016/j.ifset.2024.103582.

22 Hoppenreijs L, Brune S, Biedendieck R, Krull R, Boom RM, Keppler JK. Exploring functionality gain for (recombinant) β-lactoglobulin through production and processing interventions. Food Bioprocess Technol. 2024:1–18. https://doi.org/10.1007/s11947-024-03414-z.

23 Hoppenreijs LJG, Annibal A, Vreeke GJC, Boom RM, Keppler JK. Food proteins from yeast-based precision fermentation: simple purification of recombinant β-lactoglobulin using polyphosphate. Food Res Int. 2024;176:113801. https://doi.org/10.1016/j.foodres.2023.113801.

24 Bongaarts JF, IFAD, UNICEF, WFP and WHO. The State of Food Security and Nutrition in the World 2020. Transforming Food Systems for Affordable Healthy Diets. Wiley Online Library; 2021.

25 UNICEF. Breastfeeding: Monitoring the Situation of Children and Women. UNICEF; 2022.

26 Bosheva M, Tokodi I, Krasnow A, Pedersen HK, Lukjancenko O, Eklund AC, et al. Infant formula with a specific blend of five human milk oligosaccharides drives the gut microbiota development and improves gut maturation markers: a randomized controlled trial. Front Nutr. 2022;9:920362. https://doi.org/10.3389/fnut.2022.920362.

27 Yart L, Wijaya AW, Lima MJ, Haller C, van der Beek EM, Carvalho RS, et al. Cellular agriculture for milk bioactive production. Nat Rev Bioeng. 2023;1(11):858–74. https://doi.org/10.1038/s44222-023-00112-x.

28 Takahashi K, Yamanaka S. Induction of pluripotent stem cells from mouse fibroblast cultures by defined factors. Cell. 2006;126(4):663–76. https://doi.org/10.1016/j.cell.2006.07.024.

29 Qu Y, Han B, Gao B, Bose S, Gong Y, Wawrowsky K, et al. Differentiation of human induced pluripotent stem cells to mammary-like organoids. Stem Cell Rep. 2017;8(2):205–15. https://doi.org/10.1016/j.stemcr.2016.12.023.

30 Sumbal J, Chiche A, Charifou E, Koledova Z, Li H. Primary mammary organoid model of lactation and involution. Front Cell Dev Biol. 2020;8:68. https://doi.org/10.3389/fcell.2020.00068.

31 Tuomisto HL. Challenges of assessing the environmental sustainability of cellular agriculture. Nat Food. 2022;3(10):801–3. https://doi.org/10.1038/s43016-022-00616-6.

Marine R.-C. Kraus
Nestlé Institute of Health Sciences
Nestlé Research
Société des Produits Nestlé S.A.
EPFL Innovation Park Bldg H
CH–1015 Lausanne, Switzerland
marine.kraus@rd.nestle.com

Published online: November 15, 2024

Szajewska H, Neu J, Shamir R, Wong G, Prentice AM (eds): Shaping the Future with Nutrition. Nestle Nutr Inst Workshop Ser. Basel, Karger, 2024, vol 100, pp 192–194 (DOI: 10.1159/000540656)

Epilogue to the "Blue Books"

For the last 4 decades, the scientific papers on human nutrition presented at the Nestlé Nutrition Workshops have been published in a Book Series well known by the health care and nutrition communities worldwide as Nestle's "Blue Books." This publication of the 100th Workshop in book form will be the last of this series.

In June 1980, the first Nestlé Nutrition Workshop (NNW), "Maternal Nutrition in Pregnancy – Eating for Two? [J Dobbing, Editor, Academic Press, 1981] was held in France, organized by Dr. Pierre Guesry, the first Medical Director of Nestlé Nutrition, Switzerland, chaired by the late John Dobbing, Professor of Child Health, University of Manchester. As Professor Dobbing described in the Preface of the first publication of a "Blue Book," "the decision was made to hold a somewhat new kind of Workshop," bringing the thought of leading medical and science authorities in papers "that set out their own attitudes towards the role of maternal nutrition, if any, in the determination of fetal and infant growth." At the time, academic meetings, publications, and compendia dedicated specifically to maternal and child nutrition were scarce, less so addressing the problem internationally, and even less so supported by the private sector.

Held at least twice yearly since then, one hundred Nestlé Nutrition Workshops have brought together renowned and distinguished clinicians, nutritionists, and scientists from related disciplines to present work on their latest research, discoveries, and advances in nutrition-related fields. The Workshops included spirited commentary and debate on these topics, reflected in the high quality of the academic papers published in the Blue Books. In 2005, with NNW 57, The Nestlé Nutrition Workshop Series was incorporated into the multiple educational initiatives of the Nestlé Nutrition Institute, as part of its effort to communicate "science for better nutrition" to its broad professional audiences. These papers were up-to-date science, often "ahead of their time," reflecting all multidisciplinary scientific and clinical aspects of nutrition. And the author roster provides a "who's who" amongst global experts that have led such progress. A complete list of the books, workshop chairs, topics, and authors can be found at: https://www.nestlenutrition-institute.org/. Thus, the Workshop Series stands as a narrative that chronicles the dynamic landscape and evolution of nutrition knowledge over the last 4 decades, particularly emphasizing maternal and infant nutrition.

The first decade of Workshops (NNWs 1–25) centered around topics on malnutrition, nutrient and micronutrient deficiencies, maternal nutrition and lactation, and emerging digestive and metabolic physiology. The '90s (NNWs 26–47) saw the emergent discussion of fetal and perinatal nutrition and its impact throughout the life cycle and the obesity epidemic. They also ushered the explosion of knowledge in the microbiota (when it was still called "microflora") and probiotics. Entry into the new millennium (NNIWs 48–66) reflected the urgency of addressing the explosion of obesity and non-communicable disease, understanding genetic mechanisms in nutrition, and the windows of opportunity to shape long-term health and nutrition outcomes. The next decade (NNIW 67–94) focused on nutrition aspects in public health, the triple burden of undernutrition, obesity, micronutrient deficiencies, the critical first 1,000 days, advances in human milk and lactation, and genetic and epigenetic mechanisms. The final years (NNIWs 95–100) reflected new trends and changes in the global nutrition landscape. The latter Workshop conversations revolved around the impact of genetics, technology, social media, artificial intelligence, the bi-directional impact of the environment and climate change on nutrition, and the need for sustainable dietary changes to maintain human health and the planet's health.

Beyond their academic significance, these 100 Workshops have had worldwide reach and broad inclusion of nutrition science and healthcare professionals. They have been held in 34 countries and on every continent. This facilitated the attendance and participation of local professionals in all regions of the world, allowing about 6,000 participants to interact directly with global leaders in nutrition. This reach was amplified by the worldwide distribution of the published Blue Books at no cost to healthcare professionals. The 100 published books of the Series remain free and available digitally on the NNI's website: https://www.nestlenutrition-institute.org/.

The NNW Blue Books reflect 4 decades of evolution in the science of nutrition and should correspondingly reflect the changes in how science is communicated and disseminated. With the emergence of new channels, technologies, and diverse audiences, it is necessary to adopt new approaches. Thus, the decision to discontinue the physical publication of this Series. The tradition of the

Workshops will continue, utilizing amplification channels that align with modern educational behavior, including various mediums such as digital video, podcasts, and concise summary booklets. These approaches align with the enduring goals of effectively disseminating scientific knowledge to a broad audience and ensuring enhanced accessibility. Publishing efforts will also continue, including the *Annales Nestlé*, a series continuously published since 1942, *The Nest*, with up-to-date practical information for health professionals in critical areas of pediatric health and nutrition, and the Proceedings and summaries of symposia in national and international Conferences. A significant portion of these publications is indexed and listed in Medline/PubMed, making them readily accessible to health and nutrition professionals. All these affirm the Nestlé Nutrition Institute's commitment to remain a leading private publisher of nutrition information globally.

None of these extraordinary accomplishments would have been possible, nor will they continue to be, without the collective dedicated effort of contributors, editors, reviewers, and staff to which Nestlé and the NNI are deeply indebted. The food and diets that support global nutrition today constitute a determining factor in both human and planetary health. We all share the responsibility towards a healthier tomorrow.

Jose M. Saavedra[1]
Associate Professor of Pediatrics
Johns Hopkins University School of Medicine

Ferdinand Haschke[2]
Professor of Pediatrics
Department of Pediatrics Paracelsus Medical University
Salzburg, Austria

[1] J.M. Saavedra is former Chief Medical Officer, Nestlé Nutrition and Chairman of the Board, Nestlé Nutrition Institute.
[2] F. Haschke is former Vice-president of Nestlé Nutrition and Founder of Nestlé Nutrition Institute

Subject Index